VMS

VISUAL MNEMONICS FOR PHARMACOLOGY

VMS

VISUAL MNEMONICS FOR PHARMACOLOGY

LAURIE L. MARBAS
Texas Tech University Health Sciences Center
Class of 2003
School of Medicine
Lubbock, Texas

JOHN W. PELLEY, PHD
Associate Professor in Cell Biology and Biochemistry
Texas Tech University HSC
School of Medicine
Lubbock, Texas

Blackwell Science

©2002 by Blackwell Science, Inc.

Editorial Offices:

Commerce Place, 350 Main Street, Malden, Massachusetts 02148, USA

Osney Mead, Oxford OX2 0EL, England

25 John Street, London WC1N 2BS, England

23 Ainslie Place, Edinburgh EH3 6AJ, Scotland

54 University Street, Carlton, Victoria 3053, Australia

Other Editorial Offices:

Blackwell Wissenschafts-Verlag GmbH, Kurfürstendamm 57, 10707 Berlin, Germany

Blackwell Science KK, MG Kodenmacho Building, 7-10 Kodenmacho Nihombashi, Chuo-ku, Tokyo 104, Japan

Iowa State University Press, A Blackwell Science Company, 2121 S. State Avenue, Ames, Iowa 50014-8300, USA

Distributors:

The Americas
Blackwell Publishing
c/o AIDC
P.O. Box 20
50 Winter Sport Lane
Williston, VT 05495-0020
(Telephone orders: 800-216-2522; fax orders: 802-864-7626)

Australia
Blackwell Science Pty, Ltd.
54 University Street
Carlton, Victoria 3053
(Telephone orders: 03-9347-0300; fax orders: 03-9349-3016)

Outside The Americas and Australia
Blackwell Science, Ltd.
c/o Marston Book Services, Ltd.
P.O. Box 269
Abingdon
Oxon OX14 4YN
England
(Telephone orders: 44-01235-465500; fax orders: 44-01235-465555)

Acquisitions: Beverly Copland
Development: Julia Casson
Production: Elissa Gershowitz
Manufacturing: Lisa Flanagan
Marketing Manager: Toni Fournier
Illustration remastering by Frank Habit
Cover design by Meral Dabcovich, Visual Perspectives
Interior design by Shawn Girsberger
Typeset by Software Services
Printed and bound by Sheridan Books

Printed in the United States of America
01 02 03 04 5 4 3 2 1

The Blackwell Science logo is a trade mark of Blackwell Science Ltd., registered at the United Kingdom Trade Marks Registry.

Library of Congress Cataloging-in-Publication Data

Marbas, Laurie L.
  Visual mnemonics for pharmacology / by Laurie L. Marbas,
    John W. Pelley.
    p. ; cm.—(Visual mnemonics series)
  ISBN 0-632-04585-X (alk. paper)
    1. Clinical pharmacology—Study and teaching. 2. Mnemonics.
I. Pelley, John W. II. Title. III. Series.
  [DNLM: 1. Pharmacology—Terminology—English. 2. Association
Learning—Terminology—English. QV 15 M312v 2001]
RM301.28 .M37 2001
615′.1′071—dc21

2001035416

CONTENTS

Notice: The indications and dosages of all drugs in this book have been recommended in the medical literature and conform to the practices of the general community. The medications described and treatment prescriptions suggested do not necessarily have specific approval by the Food and Drug Administration for use in the diseases and dosages for which they are recommended. The package insert for each drug should be consulted for use and dosage as approved by the FDA. Because standards for usage change, it is advisable to keep abreast of revised recommendations, particularly those concerning new drugs.

PREFACE

Visual Mnemonics for Pharmacology is a study tool that will help you to quickly learn and memorize material presented in Pharmacology. It is visual because much of our memory is created from images, and it is mnemonic because it is constructed to aid rapid recall on examinations. Two significant features of *Visual Mnemonics for Pharmacology* are the use of humor and exaggeration, both of which are well established as memory tools, and the use of connections as an aid to integrative learning. The results you can expect are long-term retention of material and an increased rate of learning. This allows you more time to study the remainder of the material that is not covered in the *Visual Mnemonics for Pharmacology* book.

These illustrations were created to assist in my own studying, because I was always short on time to efficiently memorize facts, and because I was frustrated when I couldn't remember them longer than the hour after the test. As a mother of three small children my time for studying is limited, and must be high yield 100% of the time. These illustrations allowed me to do that, and judging from their requests for copies, it worked for many of my classmates also. Several of them stated to me that their grades improved 10 points from one exam to the next largely due to the extra study time they had gained. Also, we all agree that the long-term retention from these illustrations is incredible compared to traditional study methods of memorizing from lists or note cards.

I have attempted to combine as many pertinent facts and functions into the illustrations as possible. This book is not meant to be a total solution to your studying, but it certainly can provide an efficient and more stimulating method of learning the material.

Here are some tips on using the pictures:

1. Look at them after you have read your class notes. This will reveal what material is deemed important in your particular curriculum and what might not be covered in these illustrations, but it won't be much.

2. Write on them, color them, redraw them, add your own drawings to them – the more these illustrations are manipulated and customized by you, the more information will be retained in long-term memory. We have provided space for you to do this.

3. Since most students rewrite notes while they study, you can also record this information in the book. It will be concise and everything will be in one place for you.

I am so happy I could share my notes with you. You're in control now, so now go ahead and learn!

ACKNOWLEDGMENTS

Throughout my medical education I have been blessed with many opportunities which I thank the Lord for everyday. A special thank you must go to my grandmother, Maxine Turner, for watching my three children while I attend school and without her none of this would have been possible. My husband, Patrick Marbas, is also deserving of a tremendous debt of gratitude for making many sacrifices for me, including driving 100 miles one-way to work everyday, so that I could attend medical school. In addition, much love to my three beautiful children, Emily, Jonathan, and Gabriel, for playing quietly while I study and giving me hugs of encouragement when I needed it the most.

Also, thank you to Dr. Pelley for not only helping me with this project, but also inspiring me with his learning and study methods. His insight enlightened me and brought forth many of the ideas incorporated into these illustrations. I would also like to say thank you to Dr. Jane Colmer-Hamood, Dr. David Straus, and Dr. Rial Rolfe for their support and encouragement.

Finally, I would like to thank Erin Case, Sheemain Asaria, Nehal Shah, and my mother, Patricia Lockridge, for their friendship and creative support throughout this project. Their encouragement has been invaluable and greatly appreciated.

CONSULTING ILLUSTRATORS

Erin Case
Texas Tech University School of Medicine
Class 2003

Nehal Shah
Texas Tech University School of Medicine
Class 2003

Sheemain Asaria
Texas Tech University School of Medicine
Class 2003

Patricia Lockridge

Cholinocepter-Activating and Cholinesterase-Inhibiting Drugs

NOTES

Direct Acting

Beth—bethanechol
Porcupine—pilocarpine
Nicotine—nicotine
Car—carbachol
ACh—acetylcholine

Indirect Acting (Acetylcholinesterase Inhibitors)

Ed—edrophonium
Neon—neostigmine
Physically—physostigmine
Pyramid—pyridostigmine
Echo—echothiophate

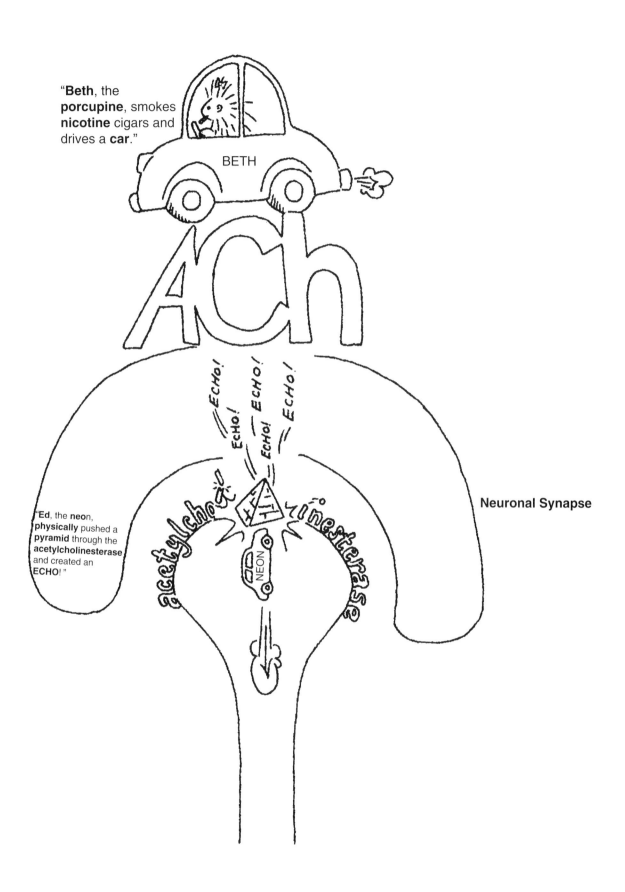

Neuronal Synapse

NOTES

CHOLINOCEPTOR BLOCKERS AND CHOLINESTERASE REGENERATORS

Muscarinic Blockers

⇒ muscles
⇒ block
- alpine: atropine is a nonselective (no muscle) muscarinic blocker
- pirate: pirenzepine is an M (one muscle) specific blocker

Cholinesterase Regenerators

PRIED the LID: Pralidoxime

Nicotinic NMJ Blockers

tuba: tubocurarine

Nicotinic Blockers

→ Nicotine
ganglionic⇒gang
hexagon: hexamethonium
Try me: trimethaphan

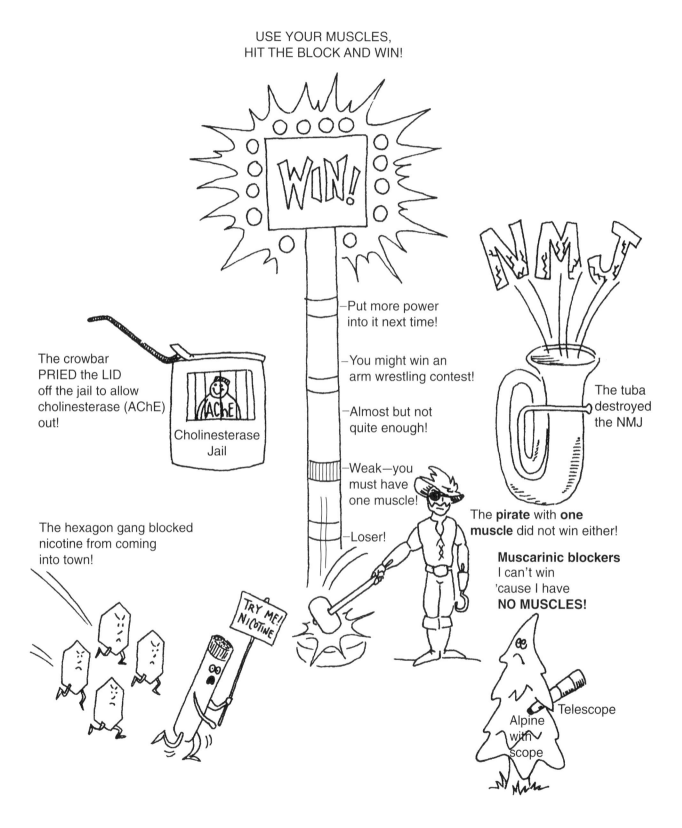

NOTES

ADRENERGIC AGONISTS

In Box

- small elephant—epinephrine
- sad coke→cocaine
  - ⇒ tricyclic antidepressants
- **TEA** tire
  - ⇒ **A**mphetamine
  - ⇒ **E**phedrine

TEA tire

T and tire⇒tyramine

E⇒Ephedrine

A⇒Amphetamine

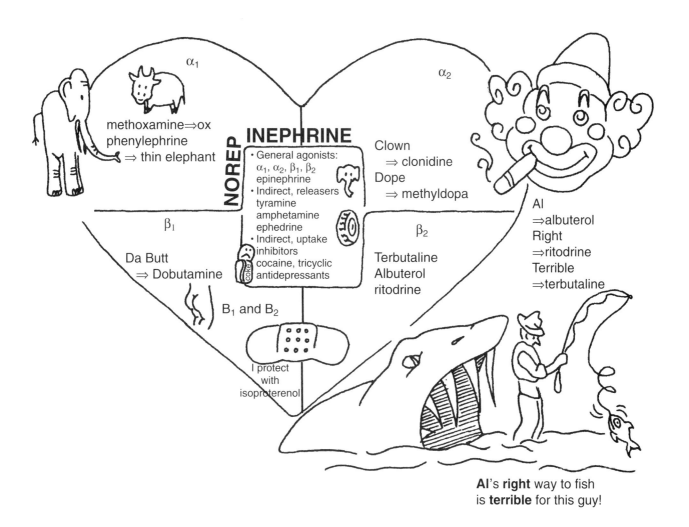

Al's **right** way to fish
is **terrible** for this guy!

NOTES

ADRENERGIC ANTAGONISTS

■ ALPHA-BLOCKERS

Nonselective

phen—phenoxybenzamine
phen—phentolamine

α_1-selective

* Prozac—prazosin
* tears—terazosin
* dots—doxazosin

α_2-selective

Yo!—yohimbine

■ BETA-BLOCKERS

Nonselective

propane—propranolol
thimble—tumolol
Nad—nadolol
α and β {carving—carvedilol
blockers {label—labetalol

β_1-selective

* ate—atenolol
* eskimo—esmolol
* meat—metaprolol

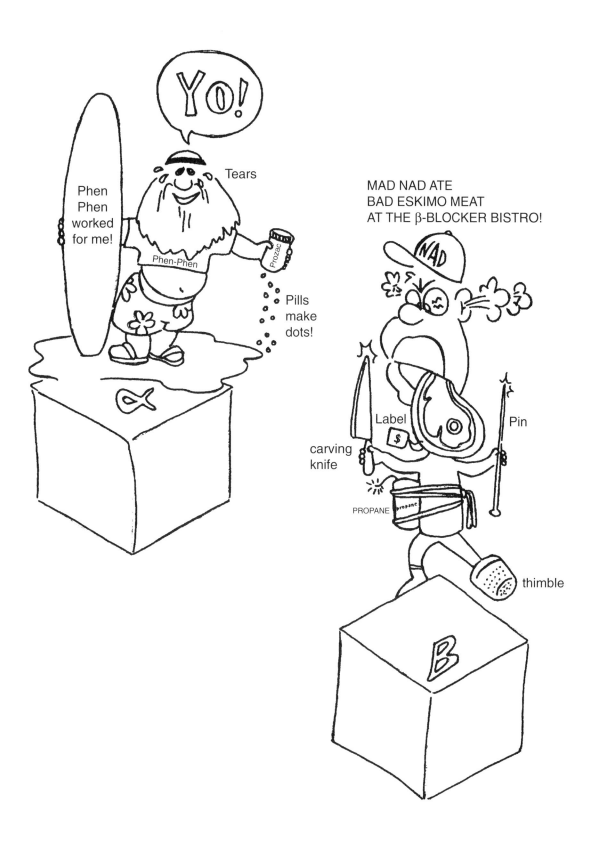

NOTES

THYROID DRUGS

T_3 and T_4 speed up metabolism giving energy and increasing body temperature.

131

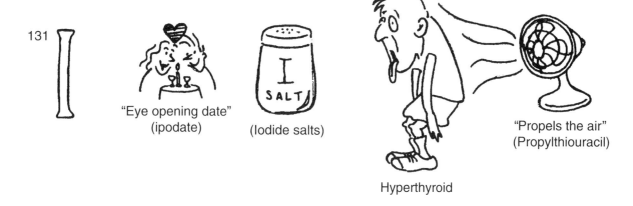

"Eye opening date"
(ipodate)

(Iodide salts)

"Propels the air"
(Propylthiouracil)

Hyperthyroid

Hypothyroid

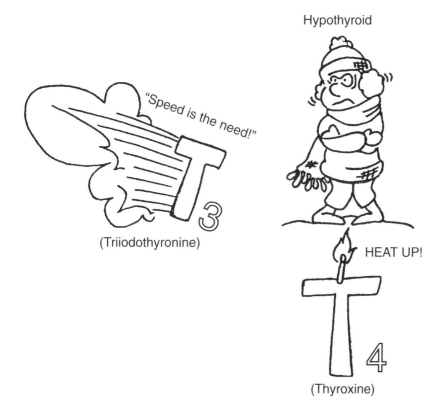

"Speed is the need!"

(Triiodothyronine)

HEAT UP!

(Thyroxine)

NOTES

IMMUNOPHARMACOLOGY—"Ig"

- drugs on "I" are immunostimulants
- drugs on "g" are immunosuppressors
- tac→**tac**rolimus
- pred→prednisone
- cyclone→cyclosporin
- BCG→↑TNF and used to treat bladder cancer

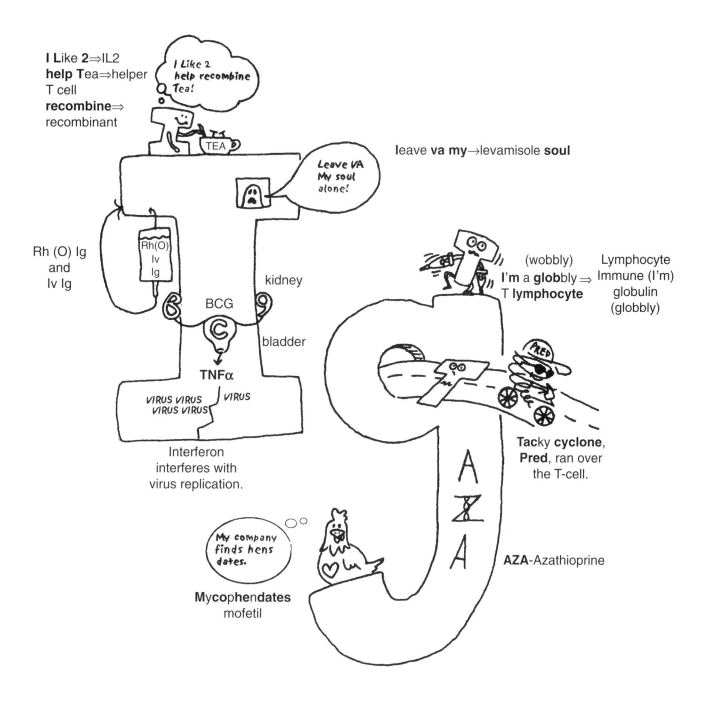

I Like 2⇒IL2
help Tea⇒helper
T cell
recombine⇒
recombinant

I Like 2 help recombine Tea!

TEA

leave va my→levamisole soul

Leave VA My soul alone!

Rh (O) Ig
and
Iv Ig

Rh(O) Iv Ig

kidney

BCG

bladder

TNFα

VIRUS VIRUS VIRUS
VIRUS VIRUS

Interferon
interferes with
virus replication.

(wobbly)   Lymphocyte
I'm a globbly ⇒ Immune (I'm)
T lymphocyte   globulin
                 (globbly)

PRED

Tacky cyclone,
Pred, ran over
the T-cell.

My company finds hens dates.

Mycophendates
mofetil

A Z A

AZA-Azathioprine

Anti-Asthma Drugs

NOTES

Ipratropium

⇒ I pray for our troops
- muscarinic antagonist

Theophylline

⇒ Theo the feline
- methylxanthine

Terbutaline (and albuterol)

⇒ terrible pain
- B_2 agonist

Zileuton and Zafirlukast

- Antileukotrienes

Beclomethasone

⇒ Become as one
- corticosteroid

Cromolyn

⇒ Cromean
- prevents release of mediators from mast cells

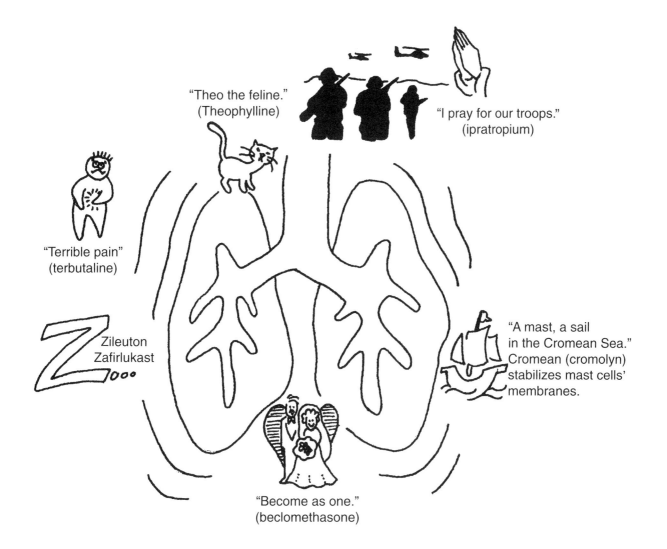

"Theo the feline." (Theophylline)

"I pray for our troops." (ipratropium)

"Terrible pain" (terbutaline)

Zileuton Zafirlukast

"A mast, a sail in the Cromean Sea." Cromean (cromolyn) stabilizes mast cells' membranes.

"Become as one." (beclomethasone)

NOTES

AUTACOIDS

H$_1$ Blockers

Chlorine—chlorpheniramine
Pros—promethazine

H$_2$ Blockers

Nizan—nizatidine
ran—ranitidine
famous—famotidine
cinemax—cimetidine

Ondansetron

⇒ on Dan sat Ron
• 5-HT$_3$ antagonist

Sumatriptan

⇒ sumo
• 5HT$_{10}$ agonist

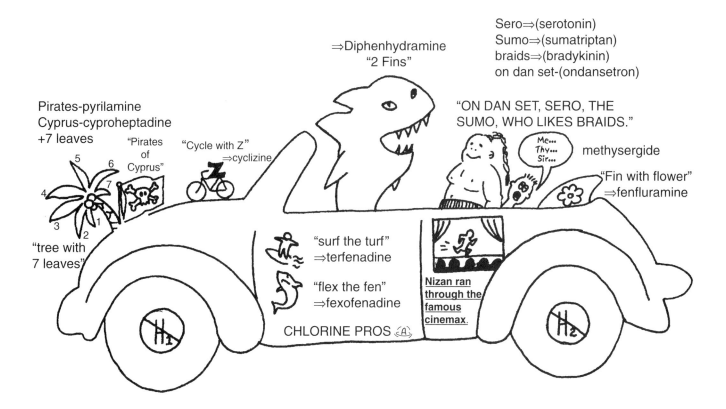

Pharmacology of GI Tract

NOTES

PHARMACOLOGY OF GI TRACT

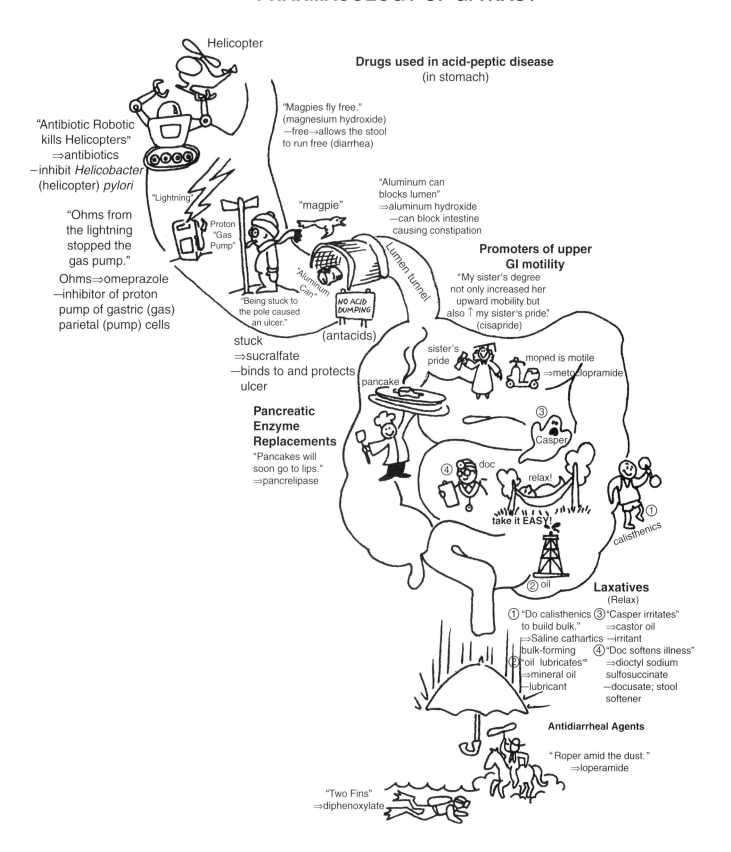

Helicopter

Drugs used in acid-peptic disease
(in stomach)

"Antibiotic Robotic kills Helicopters"
⇒antibiotics
—inhibit *Helicobacter* (helicopter) *pylori*

"Magpies fly free."
(magnesium hydroxide)
—free→allows the stool to run free (diarrhea)

"Aluminum can blocks lumen"
⇒aluminum hydroxide
—can block intestine causing constipation

"Ohms from the lightning stopped the gas pump."

Ohms⇒omeprazole
—inhibitor of proton pump of gastric (gas) parietal (pump) cells

"Lightning"

Proton "Gas Pump"

"magpie"

Lumen tunnel

Promoters of upper GI motility
"My sister's degree not only increased her upward mobility but also ↑ my sister's pride."
(cisapride)

"Aluminum Can"

NO ACID DUMPING

"Being stuck to the pole caused an ulcer."

stuck
⇒sucralfate
—binds to and protects ulcer

(antacids)

sister's pride

moped is motile
⇒metoclopramide

Pancreatic Enzyme Replacements
"Pancakes will soon go to lips."
⇒pancrelipase

pancake

③ Casper

④ doc

relax!

take it EASY!

① calisthenics

② oil

Laxatives
(Relax)

① "Do calisthenics to build bulk."
⊢⇒Saline cathartics
bulk-forming

② "oil lubricates"
⇒mineral oil
⊢lubricant

③ "Casper irritates"
⇒castor oil
—irritant

④ "Doc softens illness"
⇒dioctyl sodium sulfosuccinate
—docusate; stool softener

Antidiarrheal Agents

"Roper amid the dust."
⇒loperamide

"Two Fins"
⇒diphenoxylate

NOTES

■ LOOP DIURETICS

• block Ca^{2+}, K^+, Na^+, and Cl^- reabsorption at thick ascending→therefore no gradient→which leads to no water reabsorption

K⁺ Sparing Diuretics

Spironolactone
• antagonizes action of aldosterone at cortical collecting duct

Osmotic Diuretics

Mannitol
• ↑GFR by ↑blood volume (net movement of fluid from interstitial fluid into circulation)

Thiazides

Acetazolamide
• inhibits carbonic anhydrase in proximal tubule therefore decreasing K^+ (K^+ binds HCO_3^-)

Metolazone and Chlorothiazide
• inhibits Na^+ reabsorption in late distal convoluted tubule therefore increasing Na^+ excretion and H_2O excretion

ANTIDIURETIC

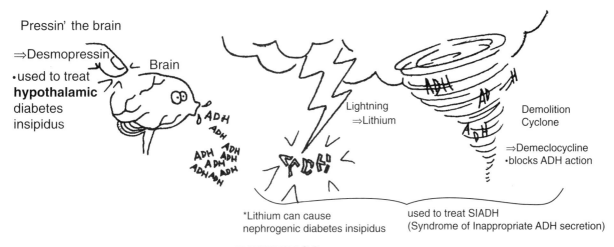

Pressin' the brain

⇒Desmopressin

• used to treat **hypothalamic** diabetes insipidus

Brain

ADH ADH ADH ADH ADH ADH ADH ADH

Lightning ⇒Lithium

Demolition Cyclone

⇒Democlocycline • blocks ADH action

*Lithium can cause nephrogenic diabetes insipidus

used to treat SIADH (Syndrome of Inappropriate ADH secretion)

DIURETICS

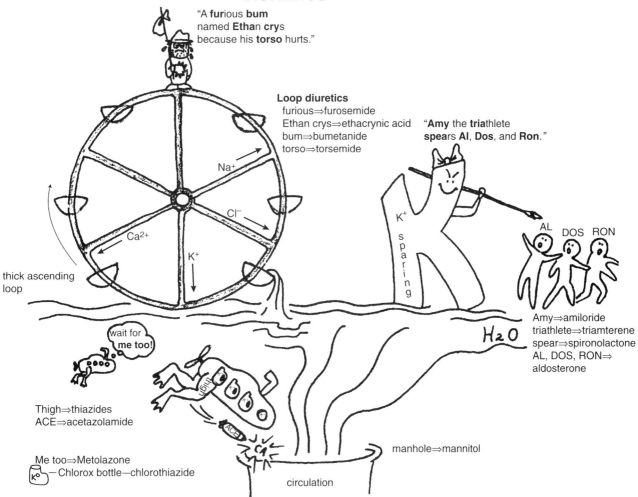

"A **fur**ious **bum** named **Etha**n **crys** because his **torso** hurts."

Loop diuretics
furious⇒furosemide
Ethan crys⇒ethacrynic acid
bum⇒bumetanide
torso⇒torsemide

"**Amy** the **tria**thlete **spea**rs **Al**, **Dos**, and **Ron**."

Na^+

Cl^-

Ca^{2+}

K^+

K^+ sparing

AL DOS RON

thick ascending loop

Amy⇒amiloride
triathlete⇒triamterene
spear⇒spironolactone
AL, DOS, RON⇒ aldosterone

H_2O

wait for **me too!**

thigh

Thigh⇒thiazides
ACE⇒acetazolamide

Me too⇒Metolazone
K^0—Chlorox bottle—chlorothiazide

ACE

CA

circulation

manhole⇒mannitol

NOTES

ANTIHYPERTENSIVES

■ DIURETICS

loop $\begin{cases} \text{furious} \Rightarrow \text{furosemide} \\ \text{Ethan crys} \Rightarrow \text{ethacrynic acid} \\ \text{bum} \Rightarrow \text{bumetanide} \end{cases}$

K^+ sparing $\lbrace$ spear $\Rightarrow$ spironolactone

thiazide-like $\begin{cases} \text{Indian purple} \Rightarrow \text{indapamide} \\ \text{chlorinated} \Rightarrow \text{chlorthalidone} \end{cases}$

thiazide $\begin{cases} \text{chlorinated } H_2O \Rightarrow \\ \text{hydrochlorothiazide} \end{cases}$

α_2-agonists

clony $\Rightarrow$ clonidine
bends $\Rightarrow$ guanabenz
face $\Rightarrow$ guanfacine
dopey $\Rightarrow$ methyldopa

Serpent $\Rightarrow$ reserpine
• prevents storage of NE
Gigi $\Rightarrow$ **gua**nethidine
• stops NE release
andrenaline $\Rightarrow$ guanadrel

β-blockers

both around word meant to remind you that these are β_1 specific
$\begin{cases} \text{NAD} \Rightarrow \text{nadolol} \\ \text{Ate} \Rightarrow \text{atenolol } (\beta_1) \\ \text{meat} \Rightarrow \text{metoprolol } (\beta_1) \end{cases}$
pin $\Rightarrow$ pindolol
propane $\Rightarrow$ propanolol
bistro $\Rightarrow$ bisoprolol (β_1)

α-blockers

tarzan $\Rightarrow$ terazosin
dots $\Rightarrow$ doxazosin
Prozac $\Rightarrow$ prazosin

Ca^{2+} channel blockers

coach $\Rightarrow$ Ca^{2+} blockers
delerious $\Rightarrow$ diltiazem
vera $\Rightarrow$ verapamil
nikes $\Rightarrow$ nifedipine

Vasodilators

Diaz $\Rightarrow$ diazoxide
miner $\Rightarrow$ minoxidil
H_2O/hydrant $\Rightarrow$ hydralazine
nitro $\Rightarrow$ nitroprusside
open the hole $\Rightarrow$ vasodilator
K's from the hose $\Rightarrow$ channel activators

Angiotensin Inhibitors

Angie $\Rightarrow$ angiotensin inhibitors
cap $\Rightarrow$ captopril
lo stump $\Rightarrow$ losartan
Linus $\Rightarrow$ lisinopril
in-a-lap $\Rightarrow$ enalapril

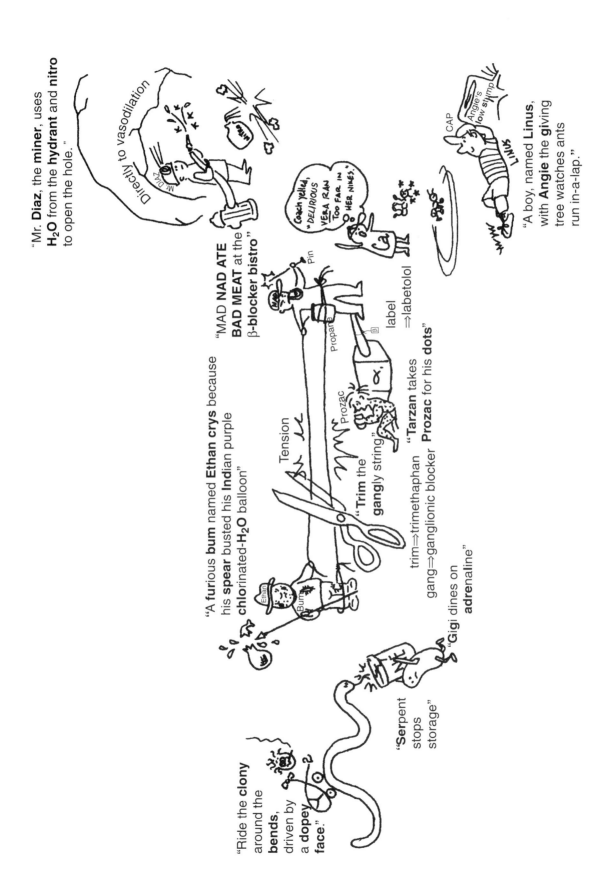

NOTES

ANTICOAGULANTS

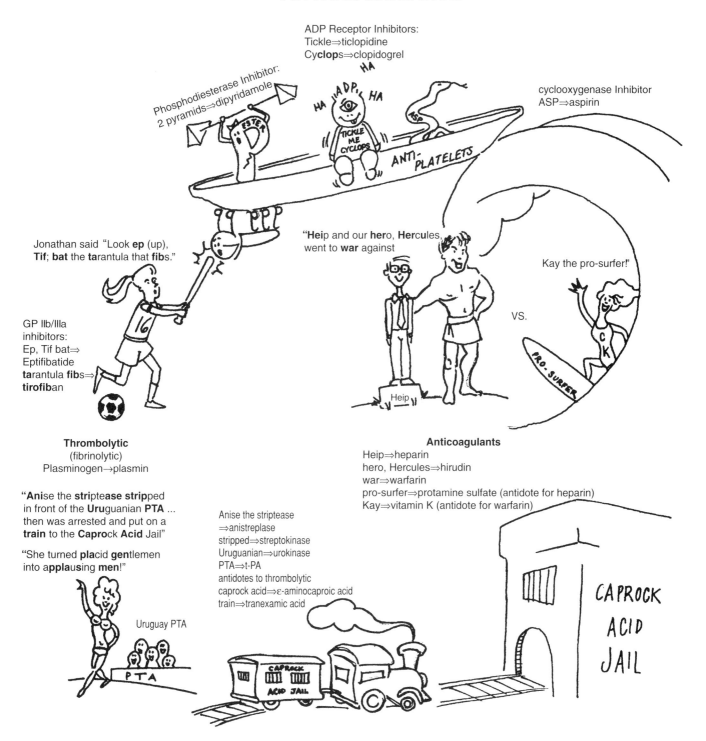

ADP Receptor Inhibitors:
Tickle⇒ticlopidine
Cyclops⇒clopidogrel

Phosphodiesterase Inhibitor:
2 pyramids⇒dipyridamole

cyclooxygenase Inhibitor
ASP⇒aspirin

Jonathan said "Look ep (up), Tif; bat the tarantula that fibs."

GP IIb/IIIa inhibitors:
Ep, Tif bat⇒ Eptifibatide
tarantula fibs⇒ tirofiban

Thrombolytic
(fibrinolytic)
Plasminogen→plasmin

"Heip and our hero, Hercules, went to war against

Kay the pro-surfer!"

Anticoagulants
Heip⇒heparin
hero, Hercules⇒hirudin
war⇒warfarin
pro-surfer⇒protamine sulfate (antidote for heparin)
Kay⇒vitamin K (antidote for warfarin)

"**Ani**se the strip**tease** strip**ped** in front of the **Uru**guanian **PTA** ... then was arrested and put on a **train** to the **Capro**ck **Acid** Jail"

"She turned **pla**cid **gent**lemen into a**pplaus**ing **men**!"

Anise the striptease
⇒anistreplase
stripped⇒streptokinase
Uruguanian⇒urokinase
PTA⇒t-PA
antidotes to thrombolytic
caprock acid⇒ε-aminocaproic acid
train⇒tranexamic acid

Uruguay PTA

NOTES

ANTIANGINAL AGENTS

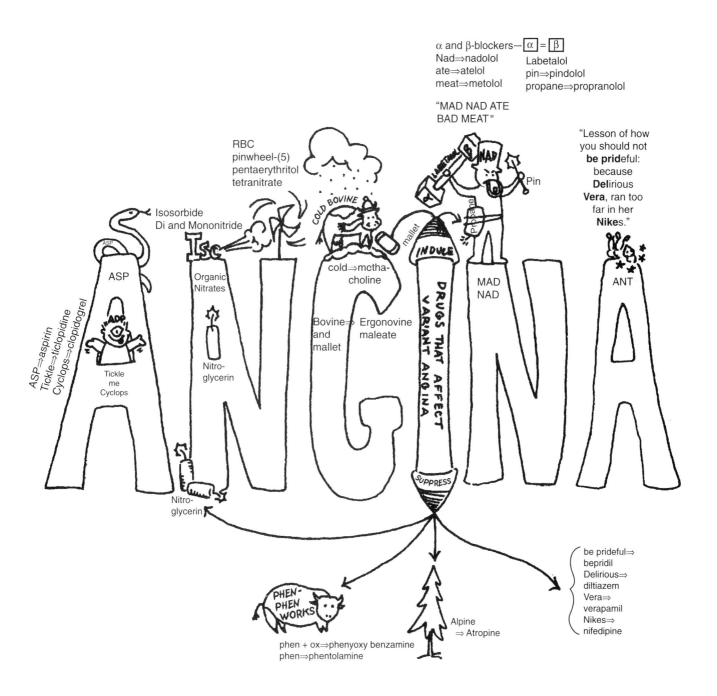

α and β-blockers— α = β
Nad⇒nadolol
ate⇒atelol   Labetalol
meat⇒metolol   pin⇒pindolol
                    propane⇒propranolol

"MAD NAD ATE
BAD MEAT"

"Lesson of how
you should not
be prideful:
because
Delirious
Vera, ran too
far in her
Nikes."

RBC
pinwheel-(5)
pentaerythritol
tetranitrate

Isosorbide
Di and Mononitride

ASP

ASP⇒aspirin
Tickle⇒ticlopidine
Cyclops⇒clopidogrel

Tickle
me
Cyclops

Organic
Nitrates

Nitro-
glycerin

cold⇒metha-
choline

Bovine⇒
and
mallet   Ergonovine
          maleate

DRUGS THAT AFFECT
VARIANT ANGINA

SUPPRESS

MAD
NAD

Pin

ANT

Nitro-
glycerin

PHEN-
PHEN
WORKS

phen + ox⇒phenyoxy benzamine
phen⇒phentolamine

Alpine
⇒ Atropine

be prideful⇒
bepridil
Delirious⇒
diltiazem
Vera⇒
verapamil
Nikes⇒
nifedipine

NOTES

HEART FAILURE

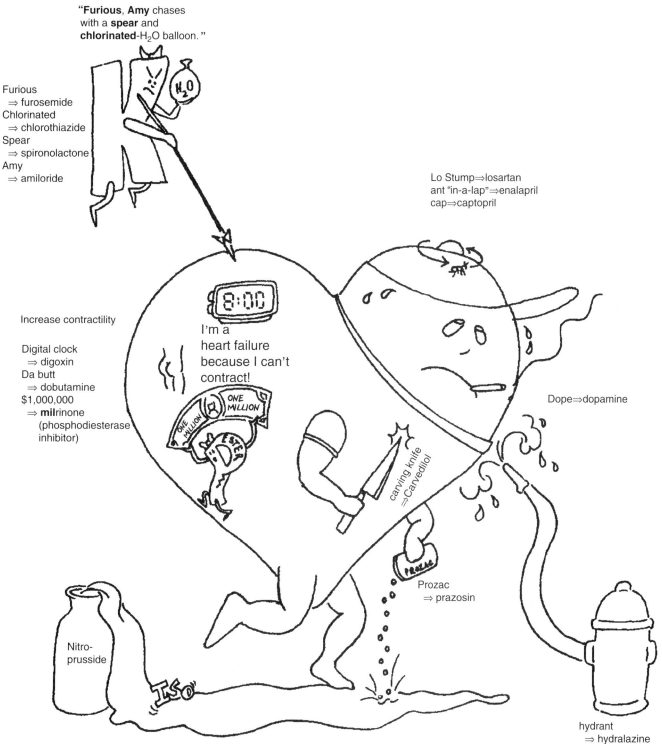

NOTES

■ CLASS IA

** slows phase $\varnothing$ depolarization
1A drugs—bind to open Na^+ channels
(which are inactivated)
2 pyramids⇒disopyramide
ℙ cane—procainamide
Skinny queen⇒quinidine
Quinidine causes:
- anorexia, hypersensitivity, thrombocytopenia, and cinchonism α-blockade (high dose)

■ CLASS IB

** shortens phase 3 repolarization
Lido⇒lidocaine
toking⇒tocainide
Mexican⇒mexiletine
pheny penny coin⇒phenytoin

■ CLASS IC

** markedly slows phase $\varnothing$ depolarization
1C flecks⇒flecainide
moric.⇒moricizine
propagates⇒propafenone

(** Indicates main mechanism of action)

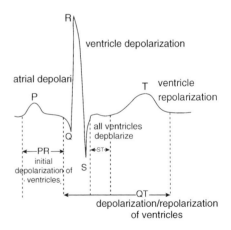

Class I (Na channel blocker)

Class IA

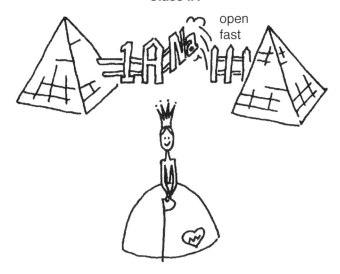

open
fast

Class IB

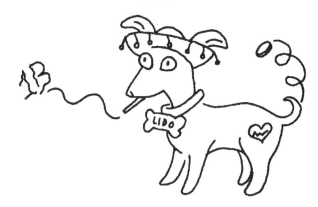

"Lido, the Mexican chihuahua
toking cocaine and tossing a pheny penny coin."

Class IC

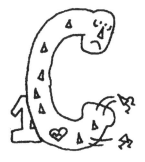

Mori C. propagates **fleck**s.

NOTES

ANTIARRHYTHMICS CONTINUED

CLASS II

** suppresses phase 4 depolarization
ace⇒acebutolol
propane⇒propranolol
eskimo⇒esmolol
block⇒β-blockers

CLASS III

** prolongs phase 3 repolarization
brety⇒bretylium tosylate NAPA
I-but⇒ibutilide
shot⇒sotalol
amigo dare⇒amiodarone

CLASS IV

** shortens action potential (AP)

CLASS V

Digitalis

Shortens refractory period in atrial and ventricular myocardial cells while prolonging ERP and ↓ conduction velocity in Purkinje cells

Adenosine

decreases conduction velocity, ↑ refractory period, ↓ automaticity in AV node

Class II (β adrenoreceptor blocker)

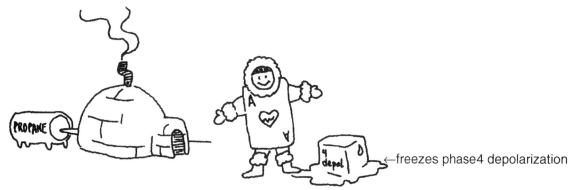

←freezes phase4 depolarization

"Ace, the **eskimo**, uses **propane** to **block** out the cold."

Class III (K⁺ channel blocker)

Class III (K$^+$ channel blocker)

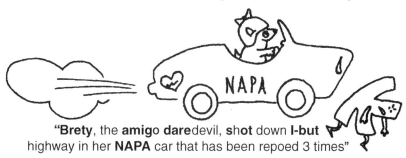

"Brety, the **amigo dare**devil, **shot** down **I-but**
highway in her **NAPA** car that has been repoed 3 times"

Class IV (Ca²⁺ channel blocker)

Class IV (Ca^{2+} channel blocker)

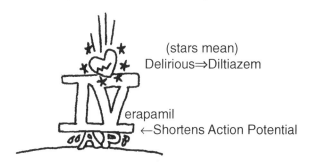

(stars mean)
Delirious⇒Diltiazem

Verapamil
←Shortens Action Potential

Class V

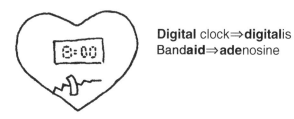

Digital clock⇒**digital**is
Band**aid**⇒**ade**nosine

Specific Arrhythmia Treatments

NOTES

SPECIFIC ARRHYTHMIA TREATMENTS

Non-sustained ventricular tachycardia or ventricular premature **complexes** (**VPC**)
- no treatment or β-blockers

Atrial fibrillation
Atrial flutter

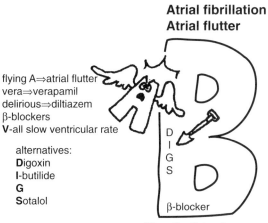

flying A⇒atrial flutter
vera⇒verapamil
delirious⇒diltiazem
β-blockers
V-all slow ventricular rate

alternatives:
Digoxin
I-butilide
G
Sotalol

β-blocker

"**Vera** the **fly**ing **A** was **delirious** after flying into the β-**blocker**, which slowed **V**era down!"

Supraventricular tachycardia

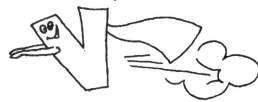

"**Super V** flew **quickly** to **aid** and **stop Vera** from hitting the ground."
Super v—supraventricular tachycardia and quickly
Aid—adenosine
Vera stop—verapamil terminates

Ventricular Fibrillation and Sustained Ventricular Tachycardia

Lido⇒lidocaine (1st)
brety⇒bretylium
amigo dare⇒amiodarone
procanine⇒procainamide

"**Lido** fell in love with **Brety**, the **pro-canine amigo dare**devil, from the **bottom of his heart**."
⇒ ventricular tachycardia

Digitalis-induced tachyarrhythmias

Digital clock spinning quickly
P⇒digoxin F₂b fragments

Torsades de pointes
(polymorphic ventricular tachycardia)

"**mag**nifying **many poin**ts on the heart "
mag⇒magnesuim
many points⇒polymorphic and de pointes

NOTES

ANTIDIABETIC

Diabetes mellitus (Type I)—autoimmune disease; pancreatic islet β cells (which produce insulin) are damaged or destroyed and can no longer make insulin

Diabetes mellitus (Type II)—due to $\downarrow$ release of insulin or $\downarrow$ response of tissue to insulin (e.g., $\downarrow$# of insulin receptors) resulting in hyperglycemia but not ketoacidosis

Diabetes insipidus—results from a deficiency of ADH (vasopressin)

Insulin

- overdosage→hypoglycemia
- $\uparrow$ glucose transport into cells (GLUT-4)
- made from beef (3 different amino acids) or pork (1 different amino acid)
- human recombinant insulin from bacteria
- factors that $\uparrow$ glucose: diazoxide, adrenergic antagonists and thyroid supplements
- factors that $\downarrow$ glucose: alcohol, weight-decreasing drugs, and catecholamine-depleting agents
- insulin resistance: 1) antibodies to insulin; 2) $\downarrow$ tissue response; 3) $\uparrow$ insulin antagonists (e.g., glucocorticoids)

Sulfonylureas (oral hypoglycemics)

- Primary mechanism of action is to stimulate endogenous insulin release
  1) Binds to ATP-sensitive K^+ channels of pancreatic β-cells→inhibition of channel→cell depolarization →activation of voltage-sensitive Ca^{2+} channels →influx Ca^{2+}→insulin release
  2) $\downarrow$ hepatic insulin CL
- orally active
- only useful to patients with some functioning β-cells

Oral hyperglycemics (Biguanides)

- do not stimulate insulin release
- $\downarrow$ intestinal uptake of glucose and $\downarrow$ hepatic production of glucose

Thiazolidinediones

- $\downarrow$ insulin resistance by binding to nuclear proliferator-activated receptors (PPARs) involved in transcription of insulin-responsive genes and regulation of adipocyte differentiation and lipid metabolism
- no effect on insulin secretion

Side Effects

- dose-related weight gain
- pioglitazone lowers serum levels of some oral contraceptives

Insulin

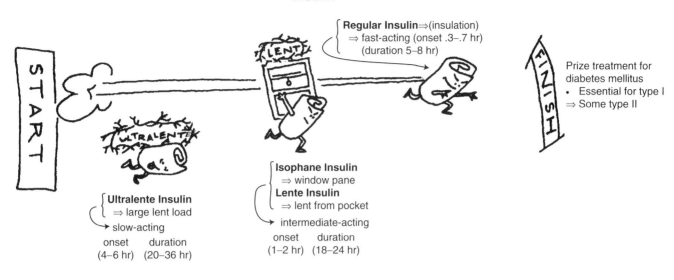

Regular Insulin⇒(insulation)
⇒ fast-acting (onset .3–.7 hr)
(duration 5–8 hr)

Prize treatment for diabetes mellitus
• Essential for type I
⇒ Some type II

Ultralente Insulin
⇒ large lent load
→ slow-acting
onset   duration
(4–6 hr)   (20–36 hr)

Isophane Insulin
⇒ window pane
Lente Insulin
⇒ lent from pocket
→ intermediate-acting
onset   duration
(1–2 hr) (18–24 hr)

Sulfonylureas (oral hypoglycemics)

Sullen Funny Family Reunion→before they broke out insulin

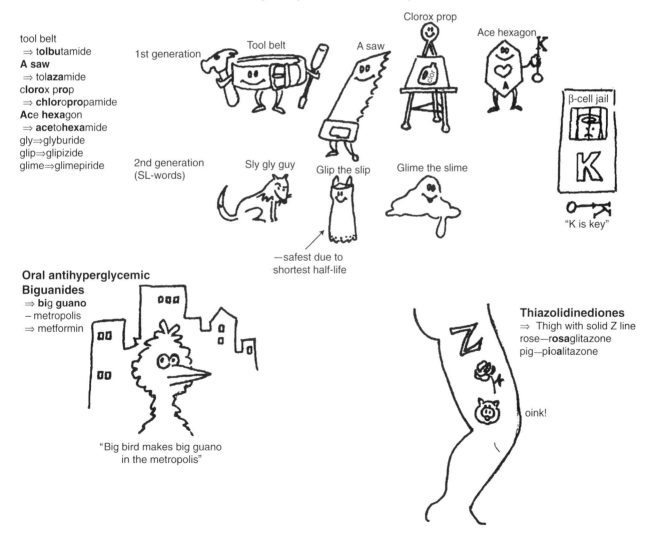

tool belt
⇒ **tolbu**tamide
A saw
⇒ tol**aza**mide
c**lorox pr**op
⇒ **chloropro**pamide
Ace hexagon
⇒ **ace**to**hexa**mide
gly⇒glyburide
glip⇒glipizide
glime⇒glimepiride

Tool belt

1st generation

A saw

Clorox prop

Ace hexagon

β-cell jail

2nd generation
(SL-words)

Sly gly guy

Glip the slip

Glime the slime

"K is key"

—safest due to
shortest half-life

Oral antihyperglycemic
Biguanides
⇒ **bi**g **guano**
– metropolis
⇒ metformin

"Big bird makes big guano
in the metropolis"

Thiazolidinediones
⇒ Thigh with solid Z line
rose—**rosa**glitazone
pig—**pio**alitazone

oink!

NOTES

ANTIDIABETIC CONTINUED

- glucagon acts by binding to a cell surface glucagon receptor that activates adenylylcyclase via a stimulatory G-protein to ↑ cAMP

Pharmacological Actions

1) ↑ hepatic carbohydrate metabolism
2) ↑ hormone release
3) cardiac stimulation

Used for:
- hypoglycemia—due to insulin overdose
- cardiovascular disease
- diagnosis
  1) glycogen storage diseases ⇒ no hyperglycemic response
  2) pheochromocytoma ⇒ pressor response
  3) insulinoma
  4) GH dysfunction

Adverse effects
- hypokalemia
- nausea and vomiting

α-Glucosidase Inhibitor

- inhibit intestinal brush border α-glucosidases→leads to decreased postrandial hyperglycemia
- Acarbose delays absorption of glucose from gut
- GI disturbances are side effects
- **A car**⇒**Acar**bose

Alpha-Glucosidase Inhibitor

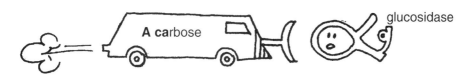

Glucagon
⇒ **glu**ts are **gon**e

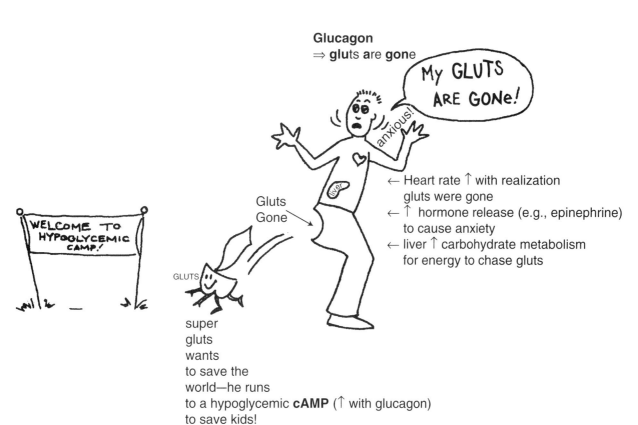

Drugs Related to Hypothalamic Pituitary Hormones

GH—Growth hormone, somatrem, somatropin

- anabolic, lipolytic, diabetogenic*
  * diabetogenic in excessive amounts or chronic administration→induces hyperglycemia
- somatomedin (IGF-1)—GH physiological mediator
- somatostatin and octreotide
  ⇒ inhibit GH release
  octreotide approved for acromegaly
  ⇒ also inhibits TSH, insulin, glucagon, serotonin, and VIP
  ⇒ also used in metastatic carcinoid, VIP-secreting tumors, AIDS-related

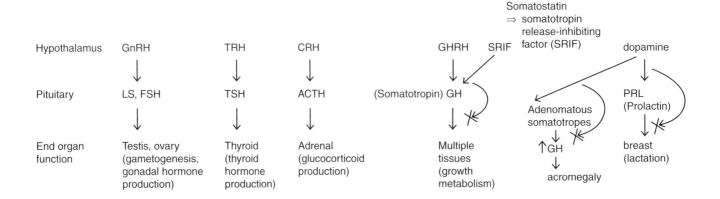

Hypothalamus	GnRH	TRH	CRH	GHRH SRIF	Somatostatin ⇒ somatotropin release-inhibiting factor (SRIF)	dopamine
Pituitary	LS, FSH	TSH	ACTH	(Somatotropin) GH	Adenomatous somatotropes	PRL (Prolactin)
End organ function	Testis, ovary (gametogenesis, gonadal hormone production)	Thyroid (thyroid hormone production)	Adrenal (glucocorticoid production)	Multiple tissues (growth metabolism)	↑GH acromegaly	breast (lactation)

NOTES

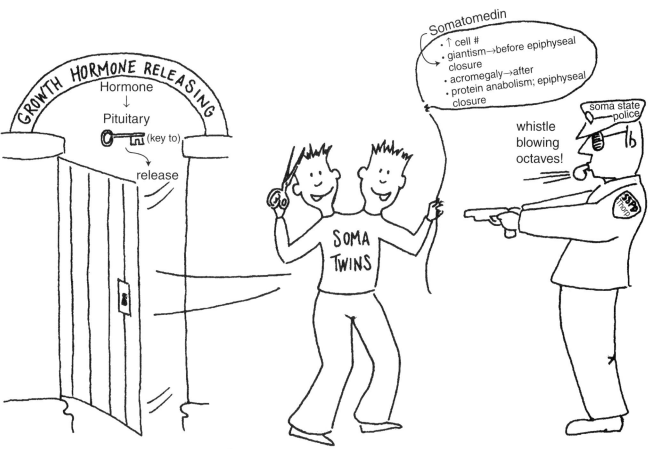

"The **trim**min' and **ropin'** **Soma** twins escaped from pituitary prison, but the **soma state** trooper blew his **octa**ve whistle and put them back."

trimmin' ⇒ somatrem
ropin' ⇒ somatropin
soma state ⇒ somastatin
octave ⇒ octreotide

NOTES

Bromocriptine and Dopamine

- both inhibit prolactin release; therefore, inhibiting lactation
- Bromocriptine used in hyperprolactemia
- don't give with medication that decrease blood pressure
- don't give to patient sensitive to ergot alkaloids

Prolactin

- lactation
- stimulates T-cells

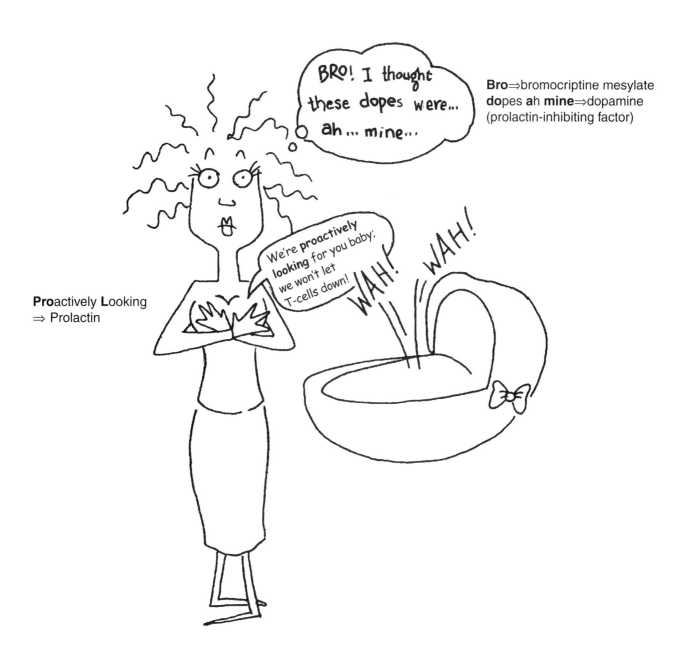

NOTES

Glucocorticoids and Mineralocorticoid Agents

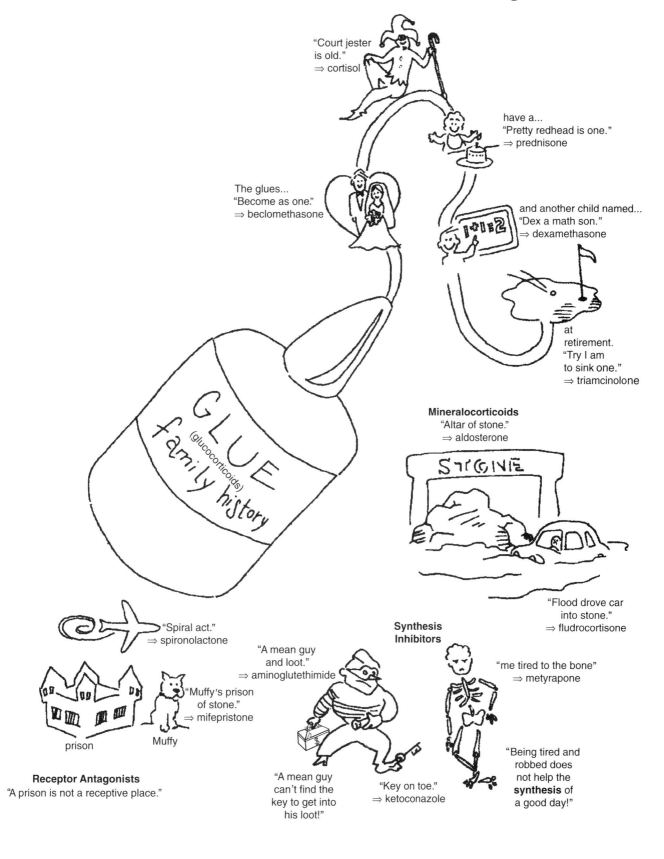

"Court jester is old."
⇒ cortisol

have a...
"Pretty redhead is one."
⇒ prednisone

The glues...
"Become as one."
⇒ beclomethasone

and another child named...
"Dex a math son."
⇒ dexamethasone

at retirement.
"Try I am to sink one."
⇒ triamcinolone

Mineralocorticoids
"Altar of stone."
⇒ aldosterone

GLUE
(glucocorticoids)
family history

"Flood drove car into stone."
⇒ fludrocortisone

"Spiral act."
⇒ spironolactone

"A mean guy and loot."
⇒ aminoglutethimide

Synthesis Inhibitors

"me tired to the bone"
⇒ metyrapone

"Muffy's prison of stone."
⇒ mifepristone

prison

Muffy

"A mean guy can't find the key to get into his loot!"

"Key on toe."
⇒ ketoconazole

"Being tired and robbed does not help the **synthesis** of a good day!"

Receptor Antagonists
"A prison is not a receptive place."

NOTES

Gonadal Hormones and Inhibitors

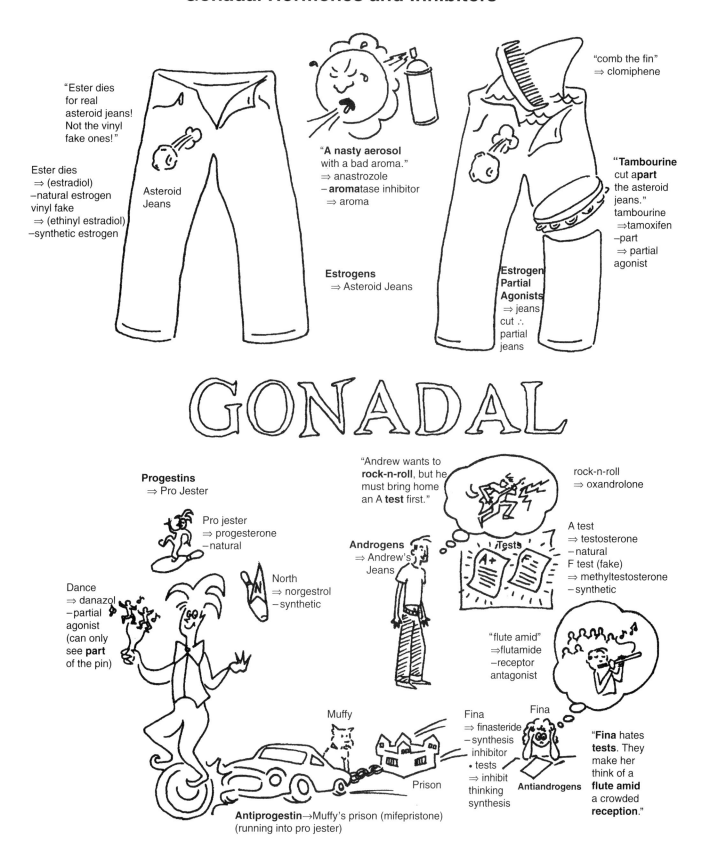

"Ester dies for real asteroid jeans! Not the vinyl fake ones!"

Ester dies
⇒ (estradiol)
–natural estrogen
vinyl fake
⇒ (ethinyl estradiol)
–synthetic estrogen

Asteroid Jeans

"**A nasty aerosol** with a bad aroma."
⇒ anastrozole
– **aroma**tase inhibitor
⇒ aroma

Estrogens
⇒ Asteroid Jeans

"comb the fin"
⇒ clomiphene

"**Tambourine** cut a**part** the asteroid jeans."
tambourine
⇒tamoxifen
–part
⇒ partial agonist

Estrogen Partial Agonists
⇒ jeans cut ∴ partial jeans

GONADAL

Progestins
⇒ Pro Jester

Pro jester
⇒ progesterone
–natural

North
⇒ norgestrol
–synthetic

Dance
⇒ danazol
–partial agonist
(can only see **part** of the pin)

Antiprogestin→Muffy's prison (mifepristone)
(running into pro jester)

Muffy

Prison

"Andrew wants to **rock-n-roll**, but he must bring home an A **test** first."

Androgens
⇒ Andrew's Jeans

rock-n-roll
⇒ oxandrolone

A test
⇒ testosterone
– natural
F test (fake)
⇒ methyltestosterone
–synthetic

"flute amid"
⇒flutamide
–receptor antagonist

Fina
⇒ finasteride
–synthesis inhibitor
• tests
⇒ inhibit thinking synthesis

Fina

Antiandrogens

"**Fina** hates **tests**. They make her think of a **flute amid** a crowded **reception**."

NOTES

DRUG THERAPY FOR ANEMIAS

foal licks acid—folic acid

"Hypochromic microcytic anemia"
ASP—ASPIRIN
BUTT ZONE—phenylbutazone
Ferry—ferrous sulfate
        ferrous gluconate (oral)
Irondex—iron-dextran (intramuscular)
Defers—deferoxamine

General

- anemia-decrease in Hb per unit volume of blood below normal
- $\downarrow O_2$ carrying capacity of blood produces hypoxia and initiates compensatory mechanisms resulting in the clinical manifestations $\Rightarrow$ tachycardia, augmented CO, $\uparrow$ BF ($\downarrow$ blood viscosity and peripheral resistance), $\uparrow$ alveolar ventilation

Bone Marrow Defects

- characterized by cytopenias in peripheral blood
- no drug treatment except for those conditions lacking hormones (e.g., hypothyroid)
- secondary marrow defects may respond to removal of substance and treatment of main infection (e.g., uremia or leukemia)

Erythropoietin

Treatment of anemia due to chronic renal failure; AIDS being treated with AZT; cancer chemotherapy; surgery

Side Effects

When used for treatment of renal disease→↑clotting in dialyzer and worsening hypertension and seizures $\Rightarrow\downarrow$erythropoietin dose

Megaloblastic Anemia

Bee
$\Rightarrow$ Vitamin B_{12} in transit factor
    $\Rightarrow$intrinsic factor

Acquired or Hereditary Hemolytic Anemias

Hereditary

spherocytic and nonspherocytic anemias, thalassemia, sickle cell
- no drug treatment except splenectomy for spherocytic type

Acquired

immune or **nonimmune**
- autoimmune hemolytic anemia, erythroblastosis fetalis, transfusion reactions

Drug Therapy for Anemias

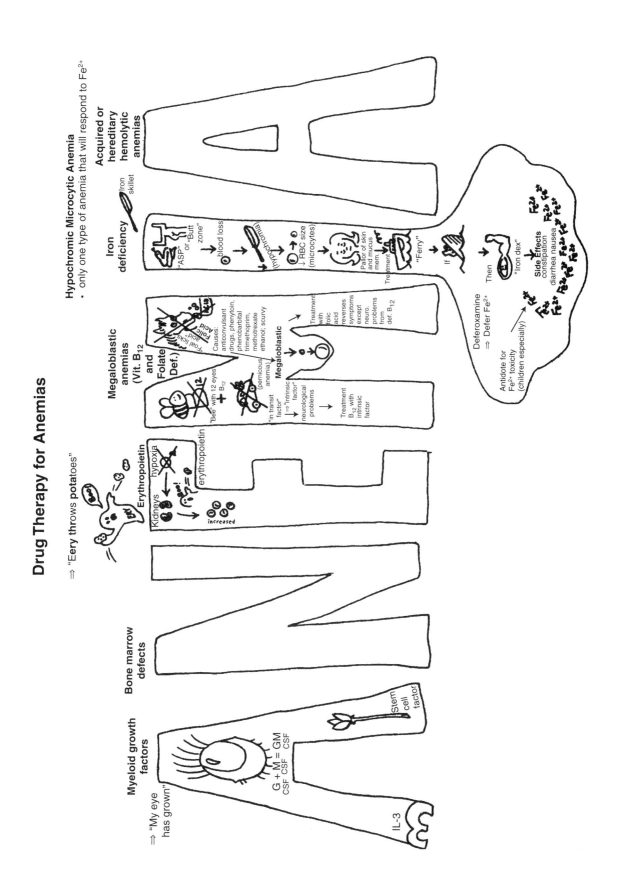

⇑ "Eery throws potatoes"

Erythropoietin

Kidneys — hypoxia — erythropoietin — increased

Bone marrow defects

Myeloid growth factors

⇑ "My eye has grown"

G + M = GM
CSF CSF CSF

IL-3

Stem cell factor

Megaloblastic anemias (Vit. B₁₂ and Folate Def.)

"Foal licks Folic Acid"

Causes: anticonvulsant drugs, phenytoin, phenobarbital, trimethoprim, methotrexate ethanol, scurvy

"Bee" with 12 eyes — B₁₂

+ (pernicious anemia) "in transit factor" B₁₂

⇒ "Intrinsic factor" ⇒ neurological problems

Megaloblastic

Treatment with folic acid reverses symptoms except neuro. problems from def. B₁₂

Treatment B₁₂ with intrinsic factor

Hypochromic Microcytic Anemia
• only one type of anemia that will respond to Fe²⁺

Iron deficiency

Iron skillet

"ASP" or "Butt zone" → blood loss → (hypochromia) → ↓ RBC size (microcytes) → Pallor of skin and mucus mem. → Treatment → "Ferry"

If → Then → "Iron dex"

Side Effects
constipation
diarrhea nausea

Deferoxamine
⇒ Defer Fe²⁺

Antidote for Fe²⁺ toxicity (children especially)

Acquired or hereditary hemolytic anemias

NOTES

Cephalosporins (cellophane ⊟)

- from mold
  1) bactericidal
  2) parenterally/orally administered
  3) side effect→hypersensitivity
- 6-ring structure

Bacitracin→Tracy's Back

1) produced by *Bacillus subtilis*
2) inhibits peptidoglycan synthesis by preventing (Tracy kicking sugar cube) the attachment of amino sugars to cell membrane lipids (♀♀)
3) bactericidal against multiplying bacteria
   - nephrotoxic⇒kidneys in back

Cycloserine

⇒ cyclone and serene

my→kills *Mycobacterium tuberculosis*
- central nervous system toxicity
- inhibits D-alanine use in synthesis of bacterial cell wall

Beta-Lactam Antimicrobial Agents

M = monobactams
⬎ = penems
CD = carbapenems
- cause seizures

Inhibitors—Administered in Combination with Beta-Lactam Antimicrobial Agents

"Tim the inhibitor, augments u in the zoo."
Tim = Timentin
augment = Augmentin
u = Unasyn
zoo = Zosyn

Penicillin

⇒ Penny
1) interferes with synthesis of peptidoglycan
   ⇒ cap on Pepsi bottle
2) binds outer cell membrane proteins
   A) carboxypeptidases⇒carbonation
   B) transpeptidases⇒traverses
3) activate autolytic enzymes
   ⇒ crack in bottle
4) bactericidal against actively multiplying cells
   G—narrow spectrum (highly potent)
   V—narrow spectrum (low potent)
   - penicilloyl—hapten responsible for hypersensitivity
   - cause GI disturbances
   - 5-ring structure
   - tolerance:
     ⇒ low MIC (minimum inhibitory concentration)
     ⇒ high MBC (minimum bactericidal concentration)
   - use low dose to stop and high dose to kill

Vancomycin

⇒ Van
amino sugars⇒mean sugar cubes
1) inhibits transfer of amino sugars to the growing end of glycopeptide on cell wall
2) bactericidal against multiplying bacteria

3) neurotoxicity—auditory nerve damage with hearing loss
   ⇒ WHAT?
- narrow spectrum

β→Beta Lactamase—resides in periplasmic space of gram-negative bacteria; degrades penicillins

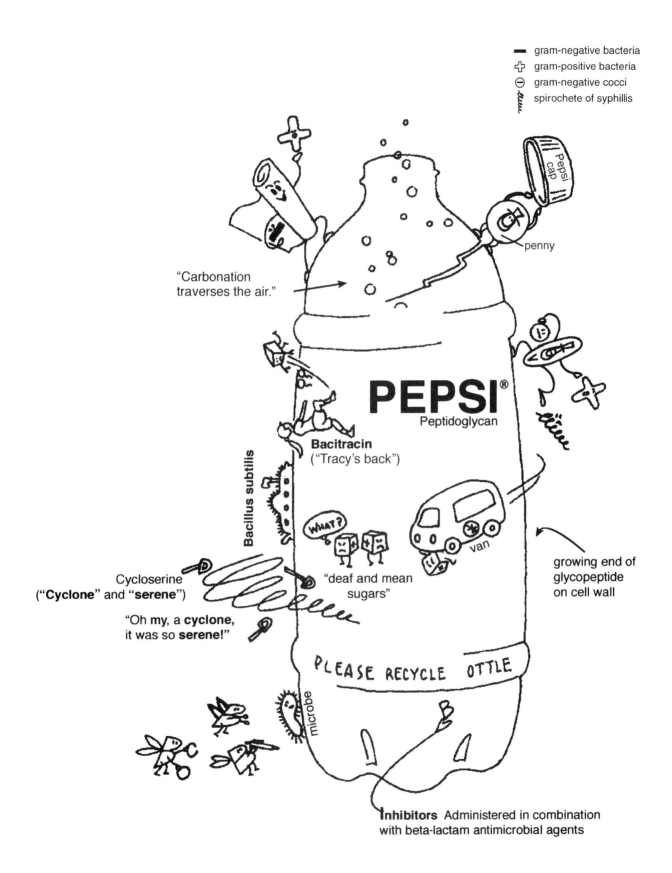

NOTES

Rifamycin

⇒ (RIF)
- inhibits bacterial DNA-dependent RNA polymerase
- broad spectrum
  ⇒ broad tombstone
- primarily used against *Mycobacterium tuberculosis*
  ⇒ TB on tombstone

Quinolone (derivative of nalidixic acid)

⇒ (**Quint**alope **alone**)⇒5 horns
- inhibits bacterial DNA gyrase
- broad spectrum (many horns)
- **enox**acin, **norflox**acin, **cip**rofloxacin
  ⇒ enox ⇒ north flock ⇒ skip
- "Enox skipped to north to join ox flock"

Metronidazole

⇒ (**Metro** runs **ni**ght and **day**!)
- MOA→4 steps
  1) passive diffusion of metronidazole into target cell
  2) metronidazole activated by reduction
  3) toxic intermediates
     ⇒ single and double strands break in DNA
  4) release of inactive end products
- narrow spectrum
  ⇒ anaerobic bacteria and anaerobic protozoa
  (*Trichomonas vaginalis*)
  ⇒ "Tricky Mona"
Side effects:
- mutagenic and carcinogenic in animals
- peripheral neuropathy
- disulfiram-like reaction with alcohol

Nalidixic Acid

⇒ (**Nal**'s—**Dixi**e)
- inhibits DNA gyrase
- narrow spectrum
  ⇒ gram-negative bacilli⇒slit ▭ in door
- used primarily in UTIs
  ⇒ outhouse means UTIs

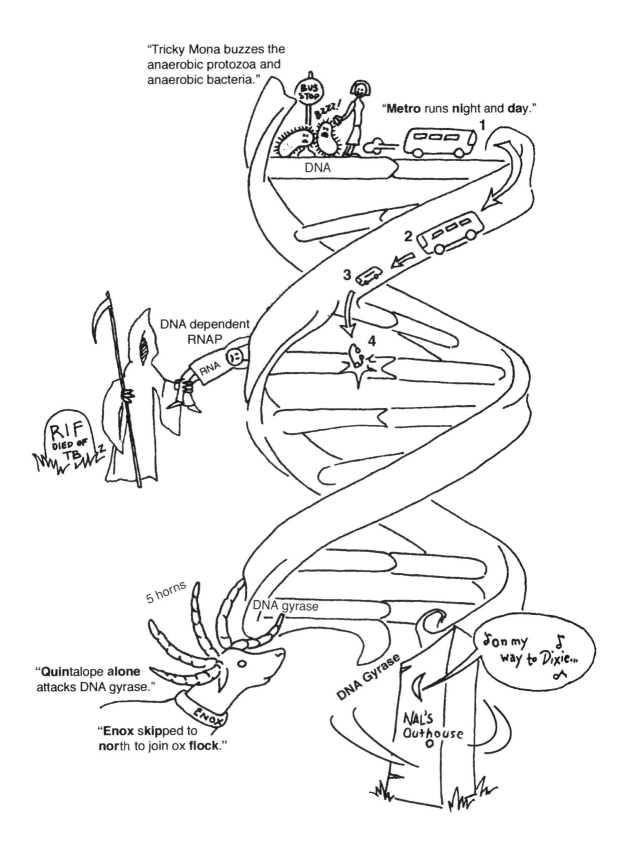

NOTES

- All bacterostatic⇒Foal licking acid

Sulfonamides

- ⇒ (SULFUR ON, AM I!)
- broad spectrum
  - ⇒ arms open wide
- used in UTIs, GI, and as topical
- structural analogs of
  p-aminobenzoic acid (PABA)
  - ⇒ (magician says "PABA CADABRA")
- inhibits tetrahydropteric acid synthetase
  - ⇒ 4 bubbles
- causes: anemia, thrombocytopenia,
  leukopenia, skin rashes

Trimethoprim

- ⇒ (**TRY MET.** IT'S **PRIME.**)
- co-trimoxazole (dog sitting on **cot**'s **rim**)
  - ⇒ mixture of trimethoprim +
    sulfamethoxazole→inhibits both steps
    of synthesis
  - ⇒ treatment of UTI, traveller's diarrhea
- competitive inhibitor of reductase
  dihydrofolate⇒"two water foals"

Sulfones

- ⇒ (cell phone)
- major agent is diaminodiphenylsulfone
  (DDS)⇒(two diamonds)
- narrow spectrum
- used in leprosy⇒(leopard)

mechanism of action of sulfonamides and
trimethoprim on metabolic pathway of
bacterial folic acid synthesis:

PABA
   ⚡ SULFONAMIDES
   ↓ (tetrahydropteroic acid synthetase)
DIHYDROFOLIC ACID
   ⚡ TRIMETHOPRIM
   ↓ (dihydrofolate reductase)
TETRAHYDROFOLIC ACID

   ↓

   purines

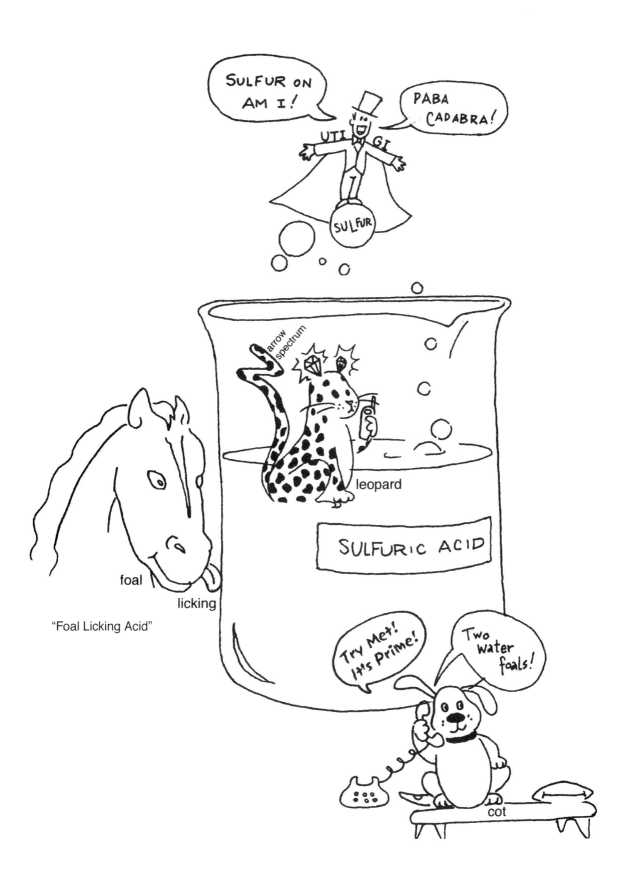

Aminoglycosides⇒"A Mean Geico Insurance Agent"

"Gentleman, Toby, and Stripper Ami sped to Kansas in a Neon."—insured by Geico gentleman—gentamicin produced by *Micromonospora*; all others by Streptomyces; treat gram positive
- irreversibly bound to 30S ((30)) subunit
- used to treat gram negative (▭)
Toby = tobramycin
stripper = streptomycin
ami = amikacin
sped = spectinomycin
Kansas = kanamycin
Neon = neomycin
Side effects:
  nephrotoxicity and ototoxicity
  ⇒ . . . WHAT?

Chloramphenicol

  ⇒ (colored fin)
- broad spectrum
  ⇒ broad range of colors
- reversibly binds 50S
- causes reversible bone marrow depression⇒bone
- causes (rarely) aplastic anemia and gray baby syndrome (premature infants lacking liver UDP-glucuronyl transferase)

Tetracyclines

C = chlortetracycline⇒Clorox bottle
D = doxycycline⇒DO$_2$x
O = oxytetracycline⇒O$_2$
M = minocycline⇒O$_2$→treatment for acne
- broad spectrum
- causes tooth discoloration⇒black tooth
- requires energy to enter cell (ATP)
  ⇒ requires energy to ride cycle
- if resistant to one tetracycline, resistant to all
- do not take with antacids because divalent cations will inhibit gut absorption of it.

Quinupristin/dalfopristin

  ⇒ (quints prison)
  ⇒ (dallas prison)
- active against gram-positive (✚)
- used in vancomycin-resistant *Enterococcus faecium* (VREF)
  ⇒ van
  and nosocomial diarrhea
  ⇒ nose with stuff running out
- hepatotoxicity side effect

Lincosamides

- lincomycin⇒links
- clindamycin
  ⇒ (clinks)
- same action as erythromycin primarily against anaerobic bacteria

Macrolides

  ⇒ (Big Mac slides)
- erythromycin⇒ERY!
- moderately broad spectrum
- binds 50S unit

"Solid Z-line"

  ⇒ (linezolid)
- inhibits on ribosomal level
- used in VREF and methicillin-resistant *Staphylococcus aureus*
- when combined with pseudoephedrine or phenylpropanolamine can cause increase in blood pressure 🚀

▭ gram-negative
✚ gram-positive
(30) 30S (Laurie is sad she is 30)
  ⇒ tRNA binds
[50] 50S (half of $1)
  ⇒ linking of growing peptide chain
(handcuffs) irreversibly bound
reversibly bound

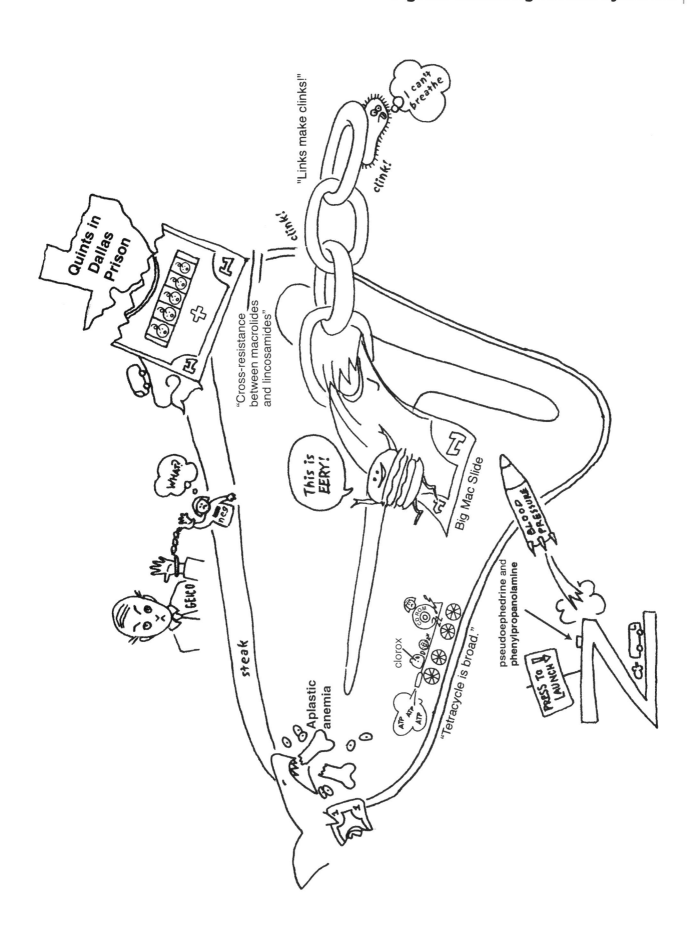

NOTES

POLYMYXIN

Poly A—toxic
Poly B
Poly C—toxic
Poly D—toxic
Poly E—same as colistin
  ⇒ (cloned)

- functions as a cationic detergent which disrupts osmotic integrity of cell membrane
- narrow spectrum of gram-negative bacilli
  ⇒ negative
- topical ointments
  ⇒ usually in combination with neomycin (neon) or bacitracin (Tracy's back)
- neurotoxic, nephrotoxic

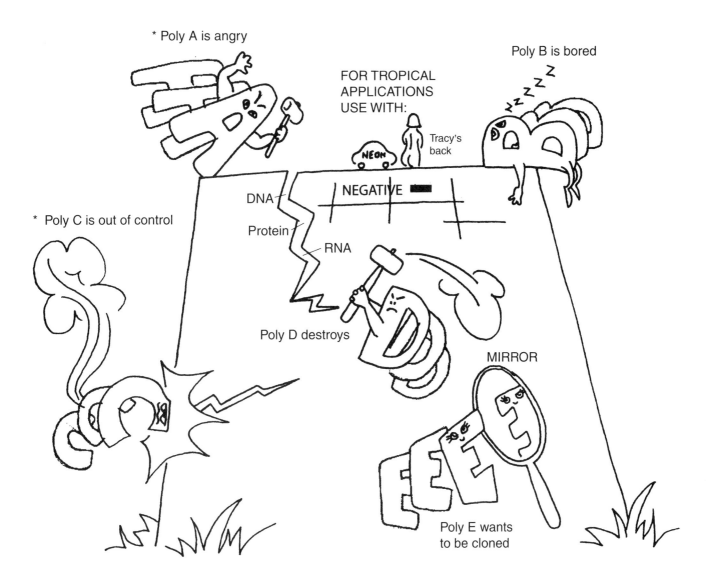

NOTES

ISONIAZID
⇒ (I saw a night alien)
- analog of B-6
  ⇒ (6 bees)
- a.k.a. pyridoxine
  ⇒ (Pirate with dots)
- treatment for *Mycobacterium* TB
  ⇒ (coughing bees)
  ⇒ (TB on pants)

NITROFURANS
⇒ nitro carrying furry ants
- used for UTIs
  ⇒ (outhouse)
- broad spectrum

ETHAMBUTOL
⇒ ET, ham, buttercup
- treatment for *Mycobacterium* TB
- rare side effects related to eyes
  ⇒ (ET's **eyes** are big)

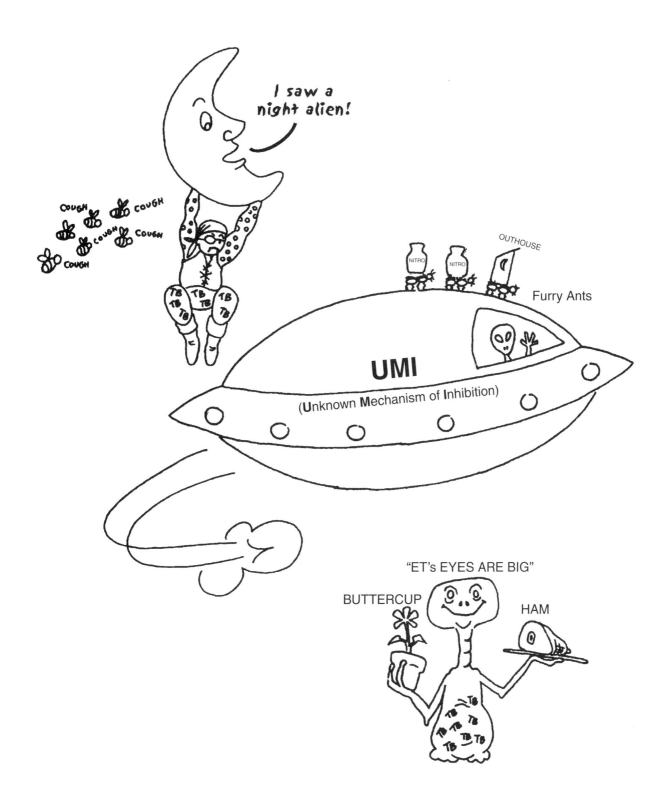

ANTIBIOTICS: PENICILLINS

Penicillinase Resistant

Methicillin⇒meth
Oxacillin⇒ox
Nafcillin⇒Naf the Knat
Cloxacillin⇒clock

Narrow Spectrum

Penicillin G
Penicillin V
• oxygen added to it
• acid stable

Broad Spectrum

Treatment for *Pseudomonas aeruginosa*

Treatment for ⎰ piperacillin⇒pipe
Klebsiella   ⎱ mezlocillin⇒Maslow's needs
Azlocillin—Azlo's Halo
Ticarcillin—Tic-Tac-Toe
Carbenicillin—carb
Amoxicillin—Am ox I!
Ampicillin—Amp
⇒ no *Klebsiella* or *P. aeruginosa*
⇒ Drug of choice for *Listeria monocytogenes*

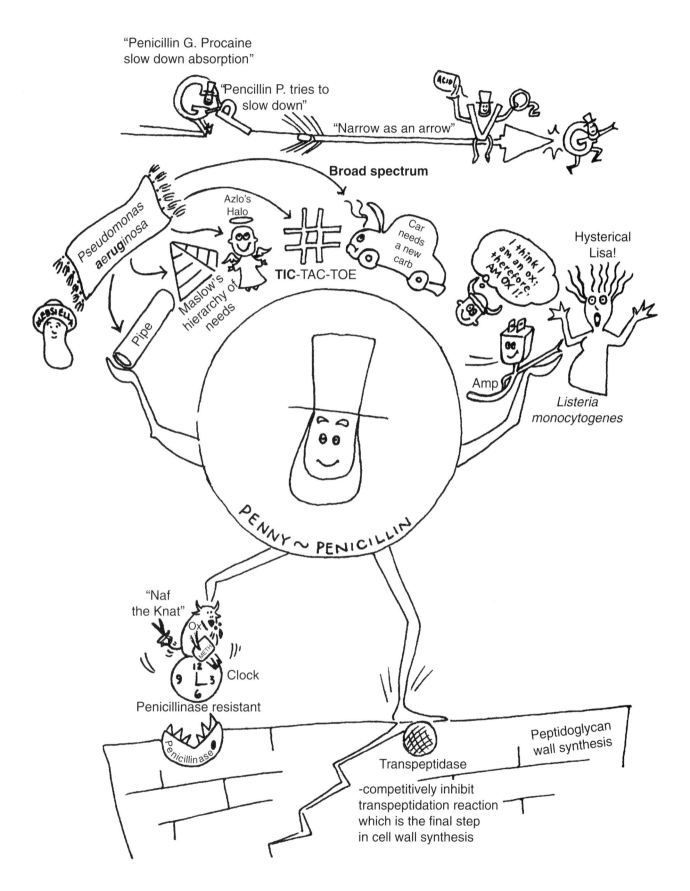

NOTES

ANTIBIOTICS I: CEPHALOSPORINS (CELLOPHANE)

**Narrow Spectrum
(1st generation)**

Cefadroxil⇒Fad
Cefazolin⇒Fazolin's
Cephalexin⇒Alex
Cephalothin⇒Thin
• 1st generation do not enter CSF

**Intermediate Spectrum
(2nd generation)**

Cefaclor⇒aclor
Cefamandole⇒a man Dole
Cefoxitin⇒fox
Cefuroxime⇒furious ox
• enter CSF

**Broad Spectrum
(3rd generation)**

Cefixime
⇒ fix me
Cefoperazone
⇒ opera zone
Cefotaxime
⇒ taxi me
• enter CSF

4th Generation

Cefepime
⇒ "Look **ep**, **I'm** 4."
• enter CSF

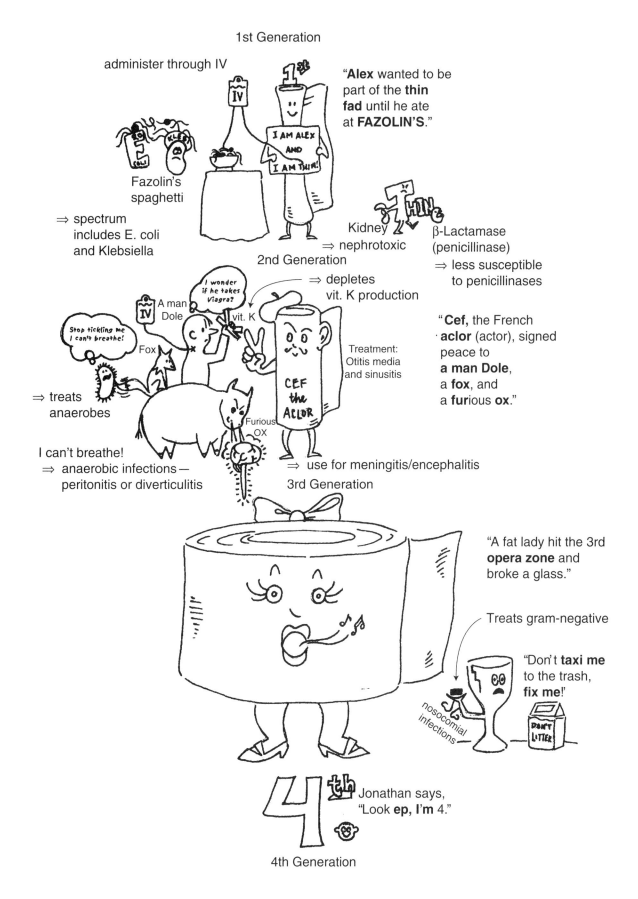

1st Generation

administer through IV

"**Alex** wanted to be part of the **thin fad** until he ate at **FAZOLIN'S**."

I AM ALEX AND I AM THIN!

Fazolin's spaghetti

⇒ spectrum includes E. coli and Klebsiella

Kidney
⇒ nephrotoxic

β-Lactamase (penicillinase)
⇒ less susceptible to penicillinases

2nd Generation

⇒ depletes vit. K production

A man Dole

I wonder if he takes Viagra?

vit. K

Stop tickling me I can't breathe!

Fox

Treatment: Otitis media and sinusitis

"**Cef,** the French aclor (actor), signed peace to **a man Dole**, a **fox**, and a **fur**ious **ox**."

⇒ treats anaerobes

Furious OX

CEF the ACLOR

I can't breathe!
⇒ anaerobic infections — peritonitis or diverticulitis

⇒ use for meningitis/encephalitis

3rd Generation

"A fat lady hit the 3rd **opera zone** and broke a glass."

Treats gram-negative

"Don't **taxi me** to the trash, **fix me**!"

nosocomial infections

DON'T LITTER

4th Jonathan says, "Look **ep,** I'm 4."

4th Generation

NOTES

■ ESTERS

Procaine
Chloroprocaine
Cocaine
Tetracaine

Cocaine

⇒ coke
• surface anesthetic for respiratory tract
• cause seizures, ↑HR, and fever
• only local anesthetic that vasoconstricts
• don't use on eye

Vasoconstrictors added with local
anesthetic to prolong stay at local site
⇒ pressing nose or squeezing tail
Norepinephrine—Norway Elephant
Phenylephrine—Aphen Elephant
Epinephrine—Jonathan (**ep** el**ep**hant)
Vasopressin—vase pressin'

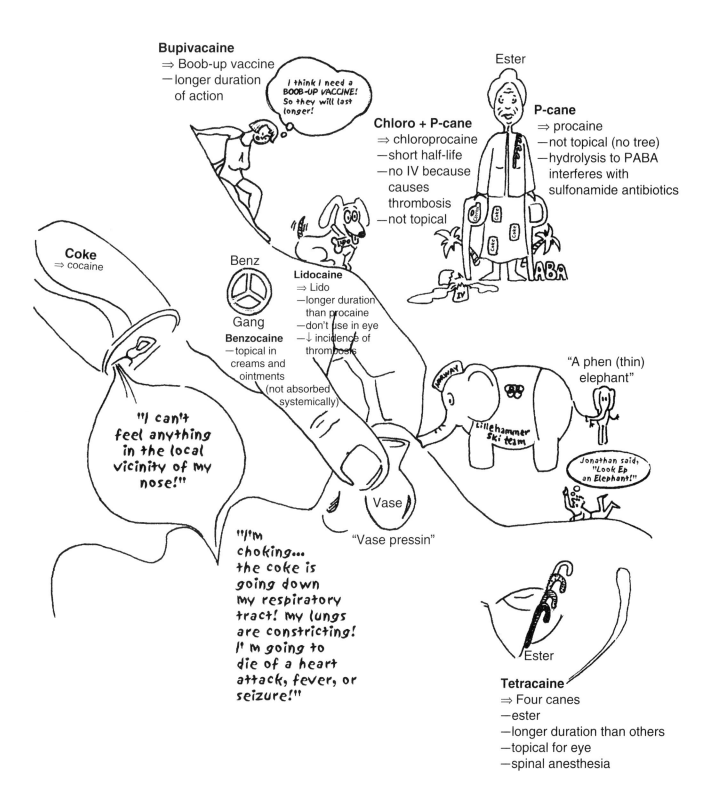

I GOT A HEADACHE!

Sumatriptan

⇒ Sumo wrestler
- acute treatment of migraine
- rebound headache more likely
- selective agonist at $5\text{-}HT_1$
  ⇒ especially $5\text{-}HT_{1B}$ and $5\text{-}HT_{1D}$
- vasoconstriction which shunts blood to brain parenchyma; block release of proinflammatory neurotransmitters
- coronary side effects most significant
- should not be used concurrently with ergot-containing compounds

Isometheptene

⇒ "I saw some heptuplets."
- sympathomimetic vasoconstrictor with acetaminophen and dichloralphenazone (mild sedative)
- Treatment for migraine
- contraindicated in: hypertension, heart disease, peripheral vascular disease

Acetaminophen

⇒ Tylenol bottle
- treatment of tension, migraine, cluster headache
- analgesic not anti-inflammatory

Methysergide

⇒ me... thy... sir...
- treatment of migraine and cluster headache
- not useful for termination of acute migraine
- serotonin antagonist
- prophylactic action due to vasodilation
- side effects: fibrosis heart, pleuropulmonary effects

Ergotamine

⇒ ergot crystal
- vasoconstrictor of both arteries and veins
- side effects: endarteritis, peripheral ischemia, thrombosis
- may cause rebound headache

Amitriptyline

⇒ Ami tripped
- antidepressant
- inhibit reuptake of norepinephrine and serotonin at nerve endings

Propranolol

⇒ propane
- Drug of choice for prophylaxis of migraine
- do not prevent cluster headaches

Lithium

⇒ Lit
- Drug of choice for cluster headache prophylaxis

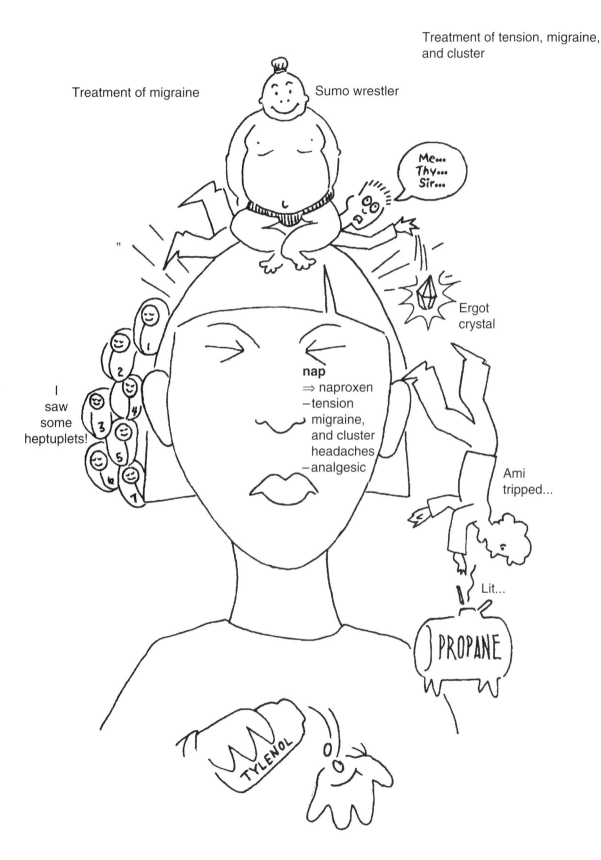

NOTES

ANTIFUNGALS

⇒ Anti fun gal

■ IMIDAZOLES AND TRIAZOLES

- inhibit CP450 and ergosterol biosynthesis

Imidazoles

Ketoconazole⇒key on toe
- topical and oral

Clotrimazole⇒clown trims
- topical

Miconazole⇒microphone
- topical and IV

Triazoles

Itraconazole⇒I train lions
- used on nails to treat fungus
- oral

Fluconazole⇒flute
- oral and IV

Econazole⇒E on engine
- inhibition of ergosterol biosynthesis
- topical treatment for dermatophytosis, pityriasis versicolor, cutaneous candidiasis

Butaconazole⇒butt with O
- treats vaginal candidiasis
- topical

Terconazole⇒turkey
- treats vaginal candidiasis
- topical

Oxiconazole⇒ox
- treats dermatophytosis
- topical

Sulconazole⇒sulking
- treats dermatophytosis
- topical

Tioconazole⇒tie with O
- treats vaginal candidiasis
- topical

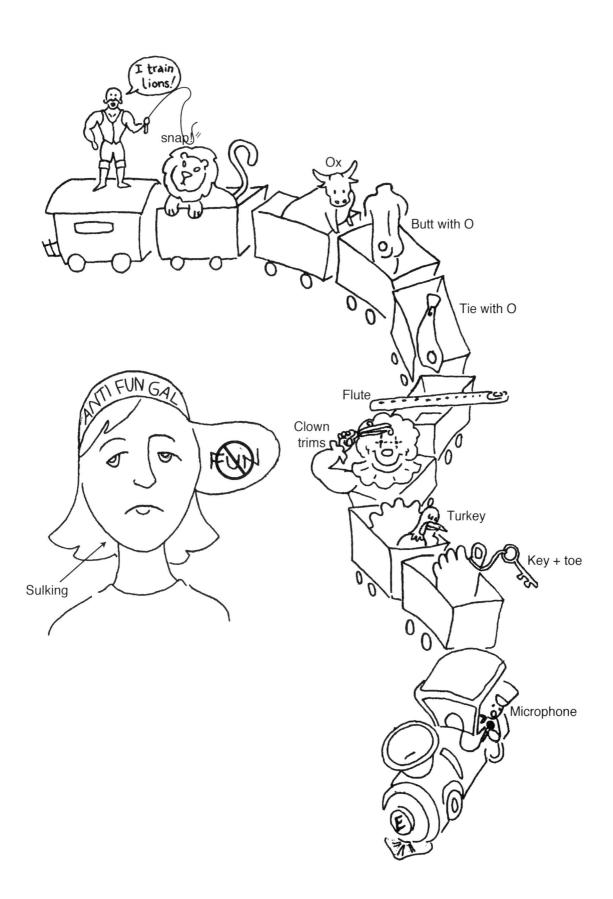

NOTES

TOPICAL ANTIFUNGALS

⇒ tropical tree

Haloprogin⇒halo and grin
- treats dermatophytosis, and cutaneous candidiasis
- prescription

Undecylenic acid and zinc undecylenate
⇒ undies and acid
- used to treat dermatophytosis such as athlete's foot
- MOA: affects fungal membrane formation and function; OTC

Ciclopirox olamine
⇒ cyclone and pie of rocks (Rox)
- treats dermatophytosis and cutaneous candidiasis
- interferes with uptake of K^+ and amino acids by fungus
- prescription

Clioquinol⇒Cleopatra
- treats dermatophytosis

Triacetin
⇒ 3 aces in tin
  - treats dermatophytosis
  - OTC

Squalene 2,3-epoxidase inhibitors⇒ "squaw leaning"
Tolnaftate⇒Toll booth
- used to treat dermatophytosis; OTC
Naftifine⇒NAFTA agreement
- used to treat dermatophytosis; prescription
Terbinafine⇒turban
- an allylamine
- used to treat dermatophytosis; prescription
Butenafine⇒**Boo ten** times!
- used to treat dermatophytosis; prescription

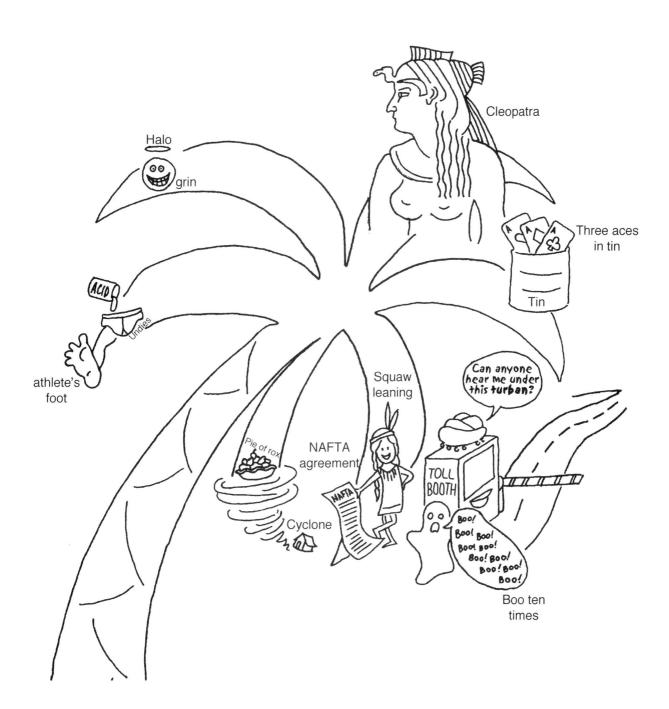

NOTES

Oral Antifungals

Griseofulvin→grizzly bear
- used for dermatophytosis
- binds to keratin and disrupts mitotic spindle, interfering with normal mitosis

5-Fluorocytosine⇒flower with 5 petals
- used for cryptococcal candida infections
- interferes with protein synthesis
- fungal resistance can develop

Echinocandin/Pneumacondin⇒ echinoderm with candy
- systemic and opportunistic infections
- B(1,3) glucan biosynthesis inhibitors

Nikkomycin Z⇒Nike symbol
- treat systemic and opportunistic infections
- inhibits chitin biosynthesis

Polyenes

Nystatin⇒N.Y. Staten Island
- topical fungicidal used to treat cutaneous candidiasis
- alters membrane function by binding ergosterol

Amphotericin B⇒amp with B on it
- used to treat systemic and opportunistic infections
- alters membrane function by binding ergosterol
- nephrotoxic
- liposomal amphotericin B complexed with lipids to increase speed of drug action and also reduces toxicity

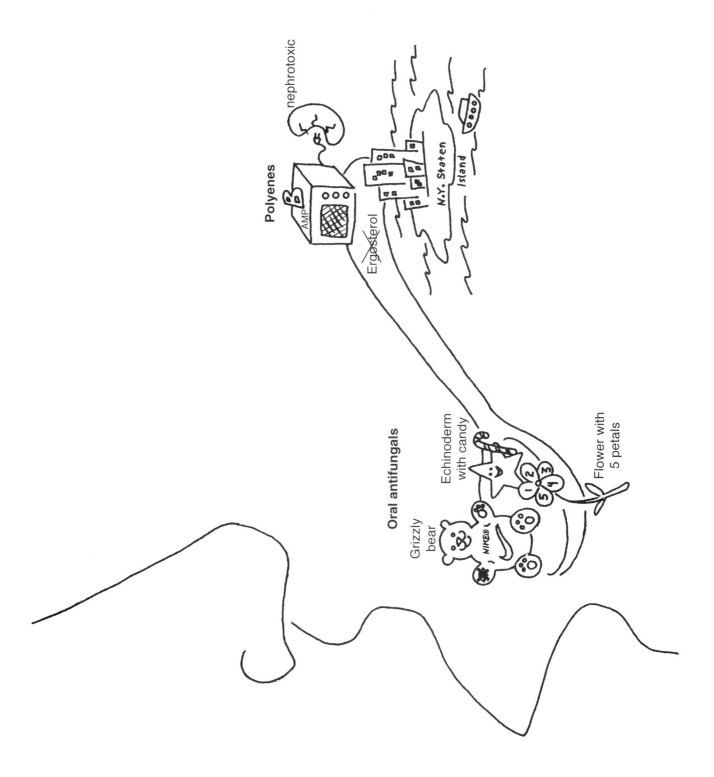

immunotherapy
- immunoglobulins:
  - ⇒ (passive vaccine): hepatitis B and A, chickenpox, rabies, measles; interferon-α-2b: HPV, HCV

Protease Inhibitors

- pharmacophores compete with viral polypeptides for the protease and bind irreversibly to it
- **indi**navir, **rit**onavir, **saq**uinavir
- MOA: prevent post-translational cleavage of GAG and GAG-Pol polypeptides that is essential for maturation of the virion: without cleavage immature non-infectious particles bud from membrane
- spectrum: HIV

Viral Reverse Transcriptase ($\frac{\bot}{H}$) Nonnucleoside Inhibitors

- ⇒ "no nuclear war"

nevirapine—"nevi→mole"
  - ⇒ MOA: binds away from **active** site of RT (**nevi is away from activist's active mouth**)

but prevents catalyst needed to incorporate base into growing chain; alters cleavage specificity of RNase H activity of RT;
- spectrum: **HIV**

Ion Channel Blockers

- amantadine→"Amen to dine"
- MOA: inhibits **M-Z** capsid protein from functioning→↑ pH (basically) of viral endosome→blocks conformational change in hemaglutinin (HA) required for fusion of membranes; prevents HA from assuming correct conformation for incorporation into budding virion
- spectrum: influenza A (fly with A wings), Parkinson's disease (causes dopamine release from intact nerve terminals)
- toxicity: slurred speech, ataxia, dizziness

Viral Reverse Transcriptase (RT) or RNA-Dependent DNA Polymerase Nucleoside Analogues

- ⇒ nuclear explosion
- **zid**ovudine⇒(AZT) (zipper): enters as prodrug→host cell phosphorylates AZT to AZT-TP→incorporated into growing DNA chain in place of thymidine-TP→ terminating it
- AZT-TP also ↓ cellular thymidine kinase so adenosine-TP levels ↓; **AZT only inhibits replication not infection**
- spectrum: HIV⇒"HIVE"

Viral DNA-Dependent DNAP Nucleoside Analogues

modified bases trick the viral DNAP into binding the analogue, which results in premature chain termination
- acyclovir (ACV) enters cell as prodrug→herpes virus thymidine kinase phosphorylates ACV→ACV-monophosphate (ACV-MP)→cellular guanosine-MP kinase→ACV-MP to ACV-TP (active)→ ACV-TP into chain→termination chain

elongation "**v**iral **h**andshake"→**HS**V-1, **HS**V-2, ⇒VZV, EBV ganciclovir→CMV
- (cretinitis in HIV patients)
- fluorouracil→HPV (genital warts)
  - ⇒ "flower with human face"

Viral DNAP, RT Inhibitors Pyrophosphate Analogues

- ⇒ "pirate hat on fox"
- bind to pyrophosphate-binding site of DNAP or RT and block dNTP binding
- foscarnet→spectrum: HIV (**hiv**e); HBV (**ham**burger); CMV (**see m**e give); HSV 1 and 2 (**h**andshake)

toxicity: can inhibit cellular DNA replication in kidney and bone marrow

Inhibition of Viral RNA or DNA Replication by Blocking Important Vital Enzymes→"Virus End"

ribavirin→"ribbon"
  - ⇒ must be phosphorylated (1, 2, or 3)
  - ⇒ ribavirin-MP→inhibits cellular **inosine** 5′ (I know sign)-5′-MP-OH→depleting GTP
  - ⇒ ribavirin-TP→interferes with 5′ capping of mRNAs by inhibiting cellular guanylyl transferase
  - ⇒ ribavirin-MP, DP, or TP→directly inhibit viral RNA-dependent RNAP

spectrum for IV—Lassa fever virus, Hantaan virus; aerosol—RSV

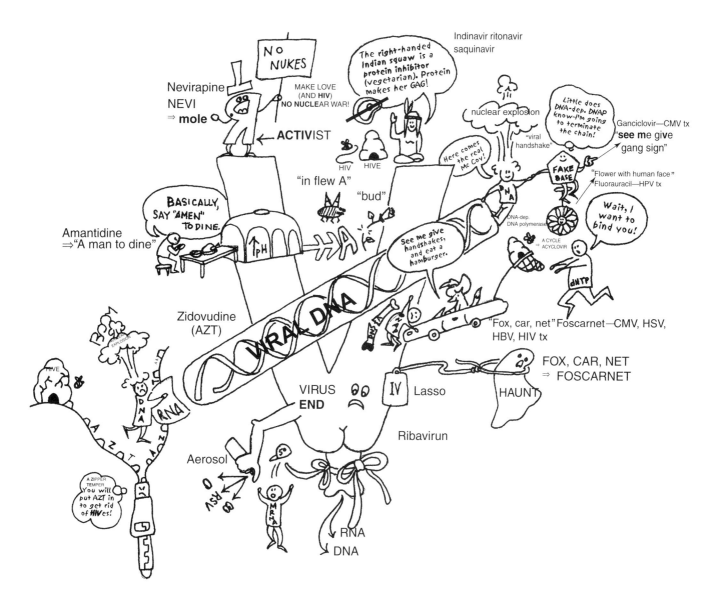

NOTES

HIV ANTIVIRAL DRUGS

⇒ hive

indian—indinavir
right—ritonavir
squaw—saquinavir

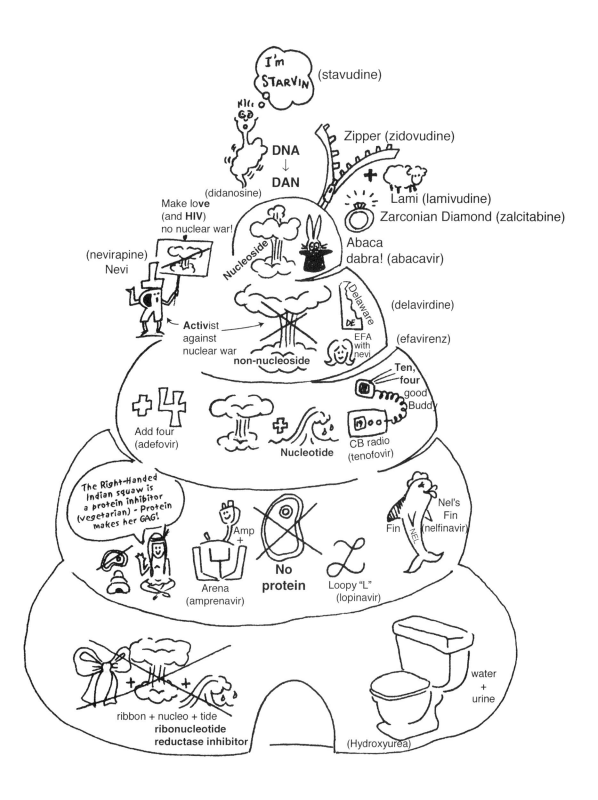

NOTES

ANTILEPROSY DRUGS

Dapsone

- absorbed in GI
- enterohepatic circulation delays excretion
- retained in tissues
- side effects: GI symptoms and blood dyscrasias

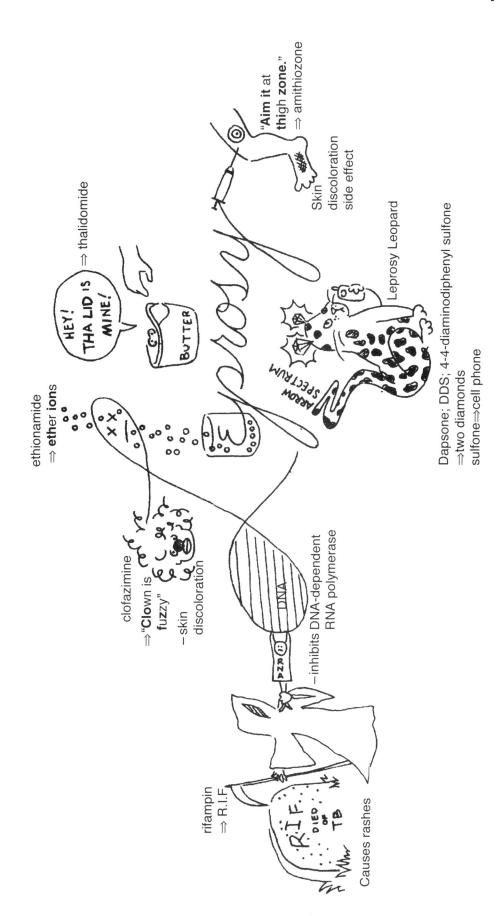

NOTES

AMEBICIDES

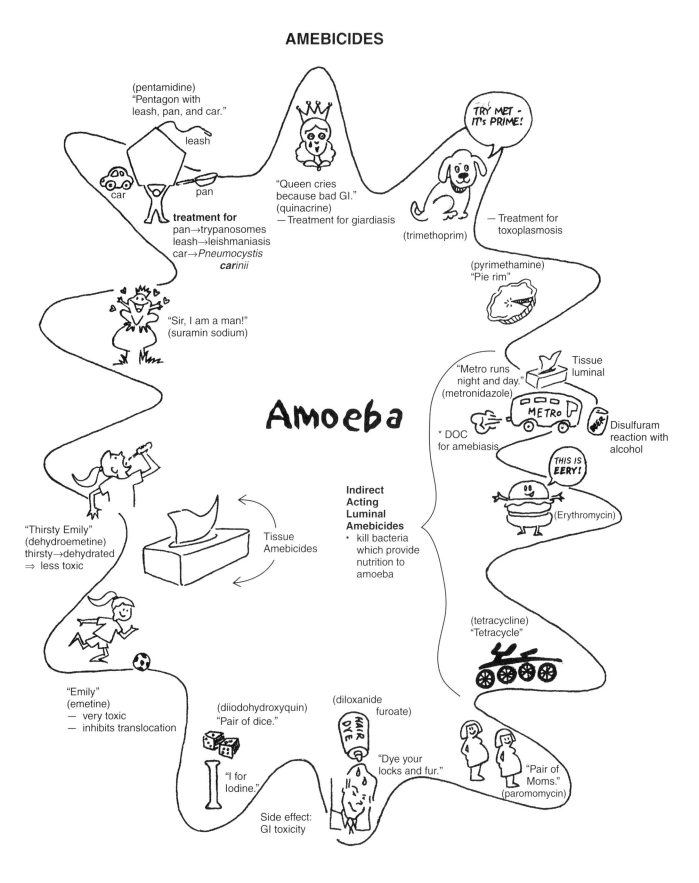

(pentamidine)
"Pentagon with leash, pan, and car."

leash

car

pan

treatment for
pan→trypanosomes
leash→leishmaniasis
car→*Pneumocystis* **car**inii

"Queen cries because bad GI."
(quinacrine)
— Treatment for giardiasis

TRY MET - IT's PRIME!

(trimethoprim)

— Treatment for toxoplasmosis

(pyrimethamine)
"Pie rim"

"Sir, I am a man!"
(suramin sodium)

"Metro runs night and day."
(metronidazole)

Tissue luminal

* DOC for amebiasis

Disulfuram reaction with alcohol

THIS IS EERY!

(Erythromycin)

Amoeba

Indirect Acting Luminal Amebicides
• kill bacteria which provide nutrition to amoeba

Tissue Amebicides

"Thirsty Emily"
(dehydroemetine)
thirsty→dehydrated
⇒ less toxic

(tetracycline)
"Tetracycle"

"Emily"
(emetine)
— very toxic
— inhibits translocation

(diiodohydroxyquin)
"Pair of dice."

(diloxanide furoate)

HAIR DYE

"Dye your locks and fur."

"Pair of Moms."
(paromomycin)

"I for Iodine."

Side effect: GI toxicity

NOTES

ANTHELMINTICS

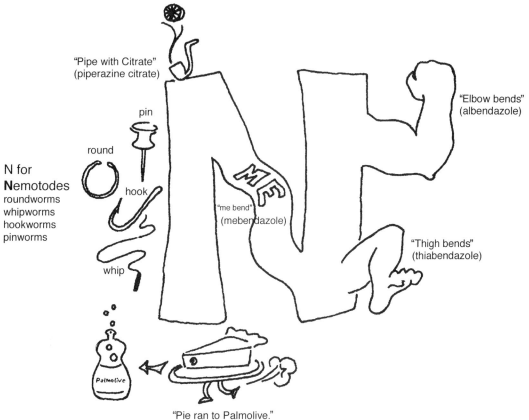

N for **N**emotodes
roundworms
whipworms
hookworms
pinworms

"Pipe with Citrate"
(piperazine citrate)

pin
round
hook
whip

"Elbow bends"
(albendazole)

"me bend"
(mebendazole)

"Thigh bends"
(thiabendazole)

Palmolive

"Pie ran to Palmolive."
(pyrantel pamoate)

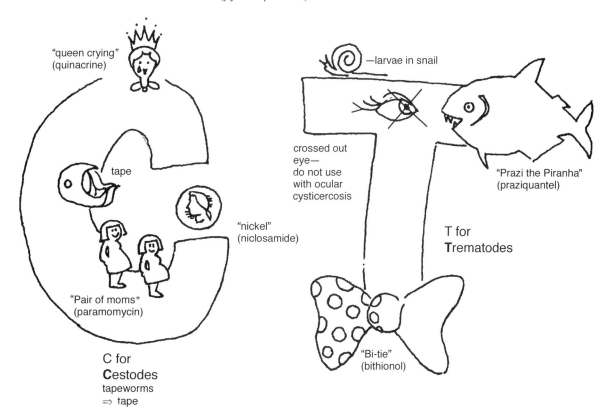

"queen crying"
(quinacrine)

tape

"nickel"
(niclosamide)

"Pair of moms"
(paramomycin)

C for **C**estodes
tapeworms
⇒ tape

—larvae in snail

crossed out
eye—
do not use
with ocular
cysticercosis

"Prazi the Piranha"
(praziquantel)

T for **T**rematodes

"Bi-tie"
(bithionol)

ANTIMALARIAL AGENTS

Plasmodium vivax
⇒ "viva"
Plasmodium ovale
⇒ "ovale"
• produce latent forms
(hypnozoites "hypnotized zoite") in the liver
which is responsible for relapses.

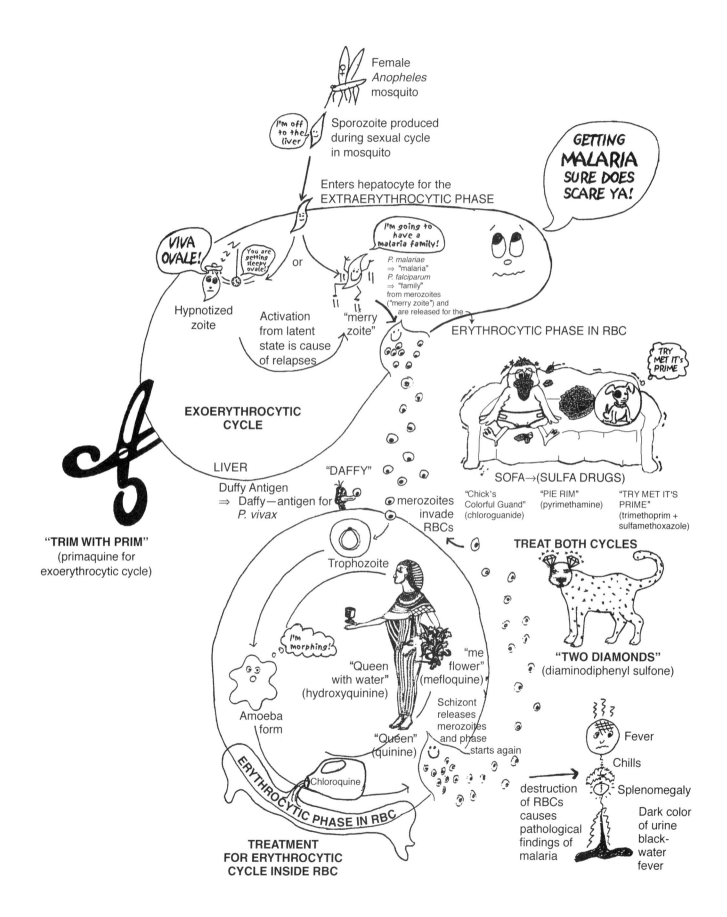

NSAIDS

■ SULINDAC

⇒ "SUE LINDA"
- Pro-drug, converted to a sulfide
- long half-life, for osteo and rheumatoid
- inhibits COX-1 more than COX-2
- side effects: GI symptoms, Stevens-Johnson

■ PENICILLAMINE

- teratogenic
- heavy metal chelator
- slows bone destruction
- serious toxicity
- long latency
- causes fever, rash, proteinuria, severe bone marrow depression
- deaths due to aplastic anemia

■ CELECOXIB

⇒ "celebrity"
- half-life = 11 hr.
- **selective COX-2 inhibitor**
- antiinflammatory, antipyretic, analgesic
- fewer GI ulcers, no ↑ in bleeding time
- protein bound, **metabolism by cyto P4502C9**
- **Inhibits cyto P450 CYP2D6,** so ↑ concentration of some β-blockers, antidepressants, antipsychotics
- Adverse: GI toxicity and pain, renal toxicity

■ PHENYLBUTAZONE

⇒ "fin on butt"
- oldest and most toxic
- potent antiinflammatory
- LETHAL agranulocytosis and aplastic anemia
- adverse effects: nephrotoxic, deafness
- used for gouty arthritis, poor for rheumatoid

■ METHOTREXATE

⇒ "Tex"—cowboy hat
- **for rheumatoid arthritis**
- **folate antagonist**
- prevents irreversible bone damage
- low dose—well tolerated
- Adverse: hepatic, bone marrow suppression, GI ulcers

■ INDOMETHACIN

⇒ Indian feather
- COX-1 and COX-2 inhibitor
- effective in rheumatoid, gouty arthritis, close patent ductus arteriosus
- adverse effects: **HEADACHE,** aplastic anemia
- avoid HTN, pregnancy

■ NAPROXEN

⇒ closed eyes mean naptime
- long half-life
- especially for **MIGRAINES**, also for rheumatoid arthritis
- well tolerated

■ GOLD

⇒ gold chain necklace
- for active rheumatoid
- stops and prevents bone and articular erosion
- protein bound, long latency
- cannot be given with penicillamine
- stop with thrombocytosis, leukopenia
- recently treatment QUESTIONED

■ IBUPROFEN

⇒ Advil
- OTC
- COX-1 and -2
- Do not use for nasal polyps, angioedema, or if there is a tendency of bronchospasticity
- **renal** toxicity

COX-1—expressed in **all tissues**
    —platelet aggregation
COX-2—only in **brain**
    —induced by cytokines

■ KETOROLAC

⇒ "**Key Toro** the bull"
- **parenteral**—strong analgesic
- potential toxicity ↑ with salicylates
- NOT for pregnancy

■ KETOPROFEN

GI and CNS effects

⇒ "Key on a Top"
- OTC
- inhibits both COX and **lipoxygenase**
- effective for rheumatoid
- does NOT alter warfarin

■ PIROXICAM

⇒ "pie on rocks"
- longest half-life (45 hr)
- effective on rheumatoid arthritis
- adverse: GI upset
- inhibits COX-1 more than COX-2

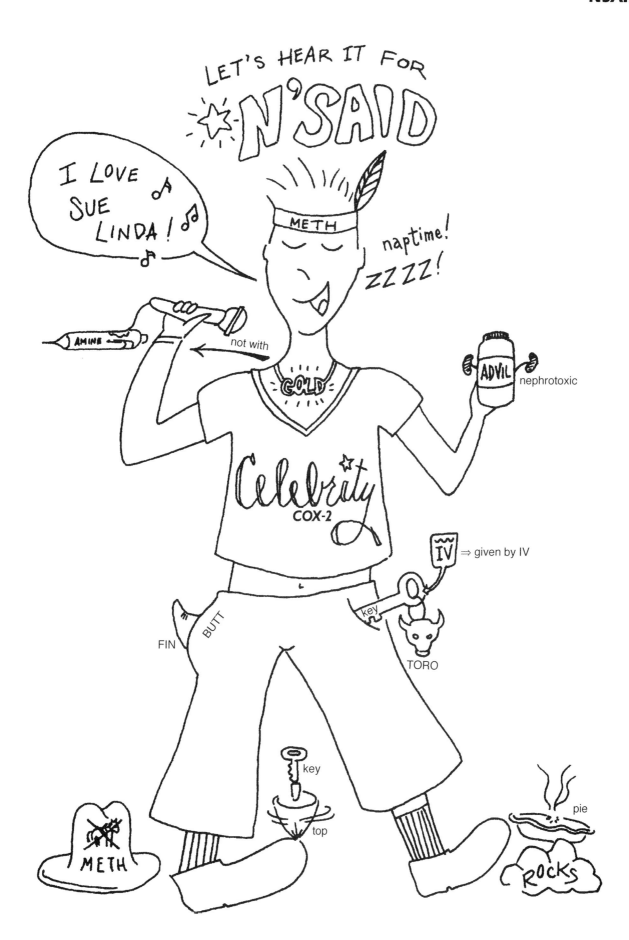

NOTES

GOUT

↑ production of uric acid
↓ excretion of uric acid
- **acute Treatment**⇒NSAIDs, colchicine, steroids, analgesics
- **long term Treatment**⇒uricosurics, allopurinol, colchicine, NSAIDs
- ↑ fluid intake to prevent stones
- ↓ weight, alcohol....
- Acute gouty arthritis: 3–10 days duration
- Chronic (tophaceous) gout
- destruction of joints, tophi form on myocardium and valves, blockage of kidney

Colchicine

⇒ "coal in chic jeans"
- binds to tubulin, inhibits phagocytes
*Antiinflammatory, only for gouty arthritis, **not** analgesic
Reserved for patients who CANNOT tolerate NSAIDs

NSAIDs/Indomethacin/Naproxen
⇒Indian   ⇒Nap

- for acute gouty arthritis
- prevent rebound attacks after cortico-steroid treatment
- used with allopurinol and uricosuric agents
*Aspirin should **NOT** be used—interferes with URIC acid EXCRETION by kidney

Allopurinol

⇒ "Aloe"
- competitive inhibitor of xanthine oxidase
- inhibits conversion of hypo- and xanthine→uric acid so **uric acid excreted**
*Gouty attacks will occur at first, since mobilizes urate from tissue stores, so USE with colchicine or NSAIDs
- TOXICITY—well tolerated **CAUTION** with kidney patients
- ↑probenecid effects

Probenecid

- inhibit reabsorption of URATE, so ↑↑excretion
- inhibits secretion of penicillin and methotrexate
- slow build-up of dose to prevent attack
- use with colchicine, NSAIDs
- avoid aspirin
  – inhibits secretion of urate

Sulfinpyrazone

⇒ "surfin' a pyramid"
*same as probenecid
- avoid aspirin
  –inhibits secretion of urate

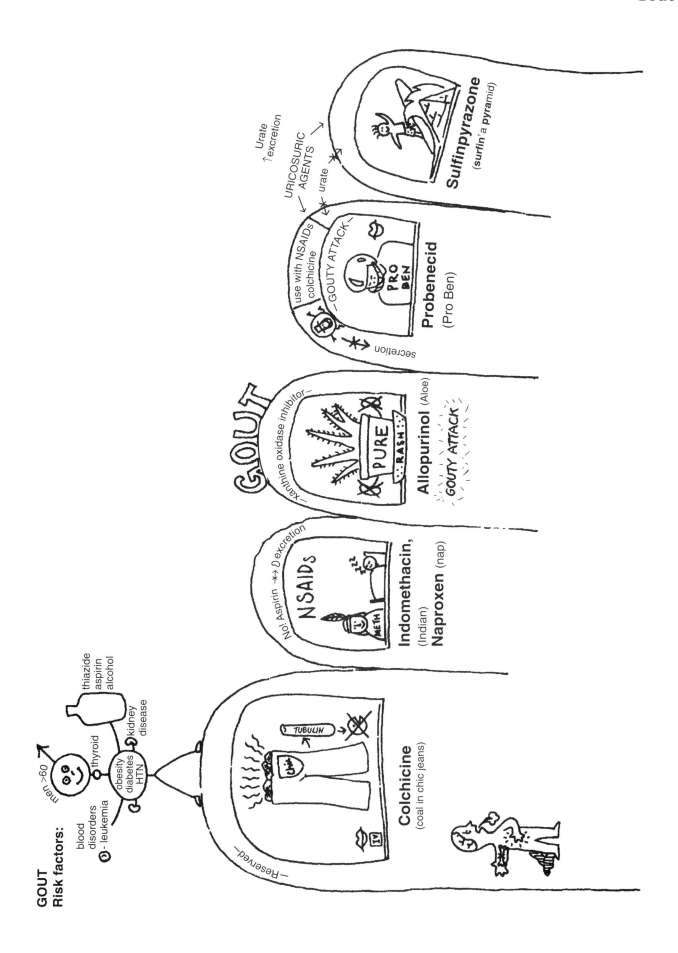

GOUT
Risk factors:

men >60
thyroid
blood disorders
⊖ - leukemia
obesity diabetes HTN
kidney disease
thiazide aspirin alcohol

Colchicine
(coal in chic jeans)

TUBULIN

—Reserved—

No! Aspirin ⟶ ↓ excretion

NSAIDs

Indomethacin, (Indian)
Naproxen (nap)

METH

G O U T

—xanthine oxidase inhibitor—

Allopurinol (Aloe)

PURE

RASH

GOUTY ATTACK

secretion

use with NSAIDs
colchicine
—GOUTY ATTACK—

PRO BEN

Probenecid
(Pro Ben)

Urate ↑excretion

URICOSURIC AGENTS

urate

Sulfinpyrazone
(surfin' a pyramid)

NOTES

HYPNOTIC/ANTIANXIETY

Pentobarbitol

⇒ "Penta Barbie doll"
Short to intermediate acting
Barbiturates: depress REM sleep
- prolong open time for Cl⁻ channels by GABA
- hypnotics are weak acids
- most are lipid-soluble→CNS
- metabolized by **hepatic microsomal** enzymes
- respiratory depression—cause of death
- **laryngospasm**—chief complaint
* since metabolized by hepatocytes
  ⇒ not for liver patients
  ⇒ many drug interactions
- used for antianxiety

Zolpidem

⇒ Z OL' ⇑⇑
- non-benzodiazepine hypnotic
- acts on GABA-A receptor (α_1)
- ↑ duration of sleep, little effect on sleep stages
- widely prescribed as hypnotic

Buspirone

⇒ "Bus on Spiral"
- Antianxiety
- little potential for abuse
- lack hypnotic and anticonvulsant properties
- No cross-tolerance or cross-dependence with benzodiazepine

Baclofen

⇒ "Back Fin"
para-chlorophenyl GABA agonist
at GABA-B receptor
- SKELETAL MUSCLE RELAXANT reduces spasm with spinal injury or MS

Benzodiazepines

- have replaced barbiturates for use in hypnosis
- depress stages 3 and 4 of non-REM sleep
- do not induce microsomal enzymes
  – lack interactions with other drugs
- NOT for pregnancy; lower abuse than barbiturates
- incidence and severity of CNS toxicity ↑ with age

Alprazolam

⇒ "Alacazam!"
- chosen for elderly
- also for antidepressant and panic disorders
- tend to develop physical dependence
  – withdraw gradually

Diazepam

⇒ Mr. Diaz in pan
- longer duration of action
- chosen for children
- is a **DOC for status epileptic**

Triazolam

⇒ Triad O' Lambs
- shortest half-life
- high rebound anxiety and insomnia
- tolerance develops quickly
  ⇒ "we tolerate ewe!"

Flumazenil

⇒ "Plume with Fumes"
- competitively ANTAGONIZES binding of benzodiazepine
- reverses sedative effects used in anesthesia
- comatose patients from large dose of benzodiazepine—regain consciousness with flumazenil
- half-life shorter than most benzodiazepines
- adverse effect: **CONVULSIONS** with patients on benzodiazepine

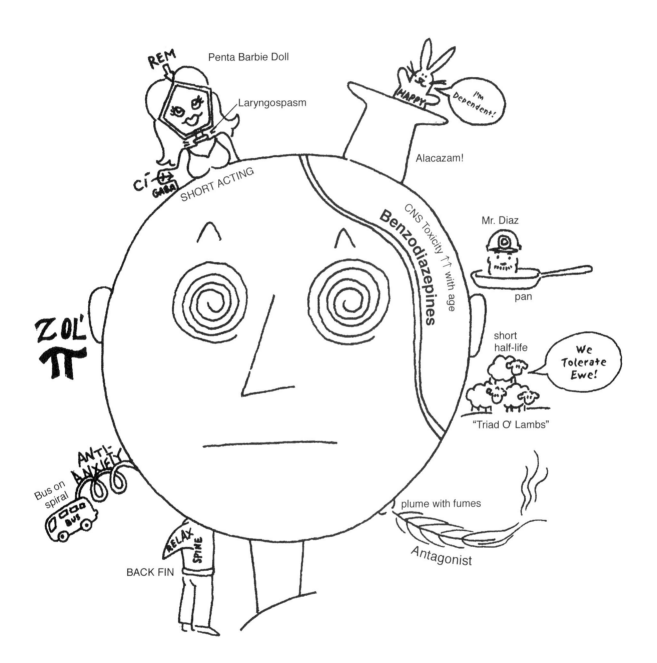

NOTES

NEONATAL/GERONTO-LOGICAL PHARMACOLOGY

■ NEONATAL

Digoxin

⇒ digital clock
• slower elimination, half-life ↑
• heart in young is insensitive to drug

Chloramphenicol

⇒ "colored fin"
• **gray baby syndrome**
• immature liver cannot conjugate drug, so ↑ serum concentration

Theophylline

⇒ THEO to cola (caffeine)
• less protein binding
• metabolized to CAFFEINE

Warfarin

⇒ WAR
• small
• crosses placenta
• teratogen

Heparin

⇒ HIEP
• large, polar
• does not cross placenta
• safer

■ GERONTOLOGICAL

Levodopa

⇒ "L on a dope"
• increased bioavailability due to ↓ stomach dopa decarboxylase activity

Warfarin

⇒ WAR
• ↓ albumin levels cause ↑ free drug
• not affected by metabolism

Procainamide

⇒ cane
• hydrophilic
• ↓ water content, ↓ BF, ↓ muscle leads to increased plasma concentration
• narrow therapeutic index so ↓ renal clearance leads to increased blood levels

Propranolol

⇒ propane
• decreased metabolism, so ↑ half-life

Diazepam

⇒ "Mr. Diaz"
• lipophilic drug
• increased storage
• decreased metabolism, so ↑ half-life

Opiates

⇒ "opal"
• increased responsiveness

GERONTOLOGICAL

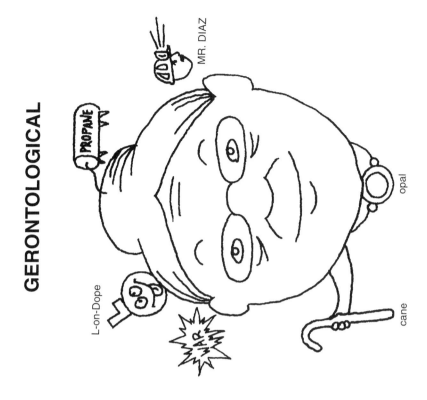

NEONATAL

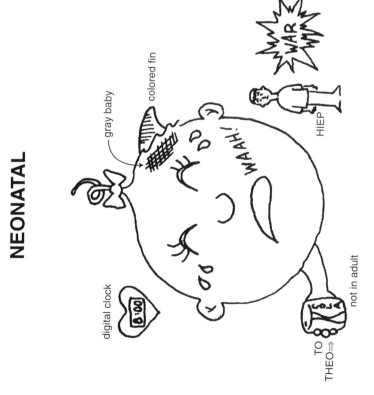

NOTES

NOTES

ANTIPSYCHOTICS

Phenothiazines

alipathic: chlorpromazine
piperidines: thioridazine
piperazines: trifluoperazine, fluphenazine
butyrophenones: haloperidol
heterocyclics: clozapine, olanzapine,
risperidone, sertindole, quetiapine

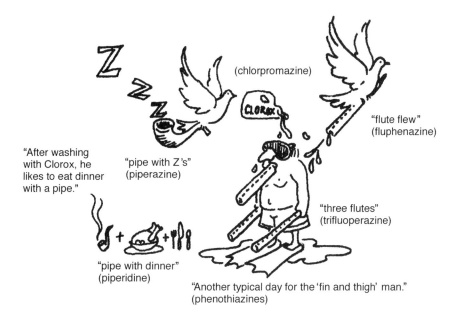

Typical Antipsychotics

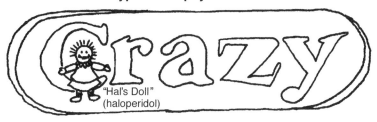

Atypical Antipsychotics

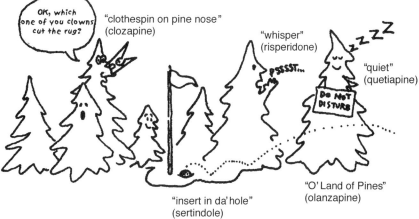

NOTES

ANTIDEPRESSANTS

1st generation

1st generation: MOA inhibitor
(tranylcypromine)
"train cycles around mind"

3rd generation

2nd generation

Desi says:
"This bra is mine!"
(desipramine)
2nd generation
tricyclic (tricycle)
antidepressants

Desi

Tricycle

"Flying ox"
(fluoxetine)
—selective serotonin reuptake inhibitor

"Pair ox heads"
(paroxetine)
—serotonin reuptake
inhibitor

"Be proper,
don't smoke
dope!"
(Bupropion)
—dopamine (dope)
uptake inhibitor

"Sir Trey
standing
in a line."
(sertraline)
—serotonin
reuptake
inhibitor

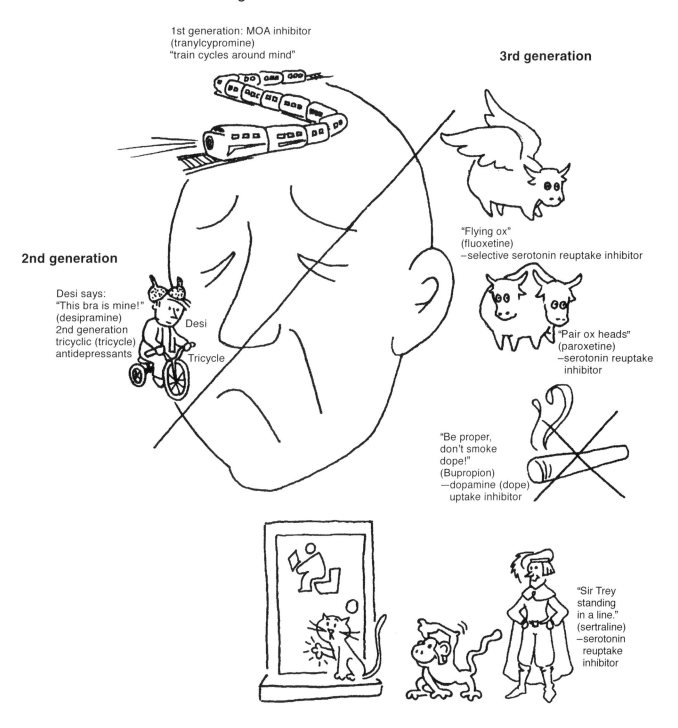

NOTES

PARKINSON'S DISEASE AND OTHER MOVEMENT DISORDERS

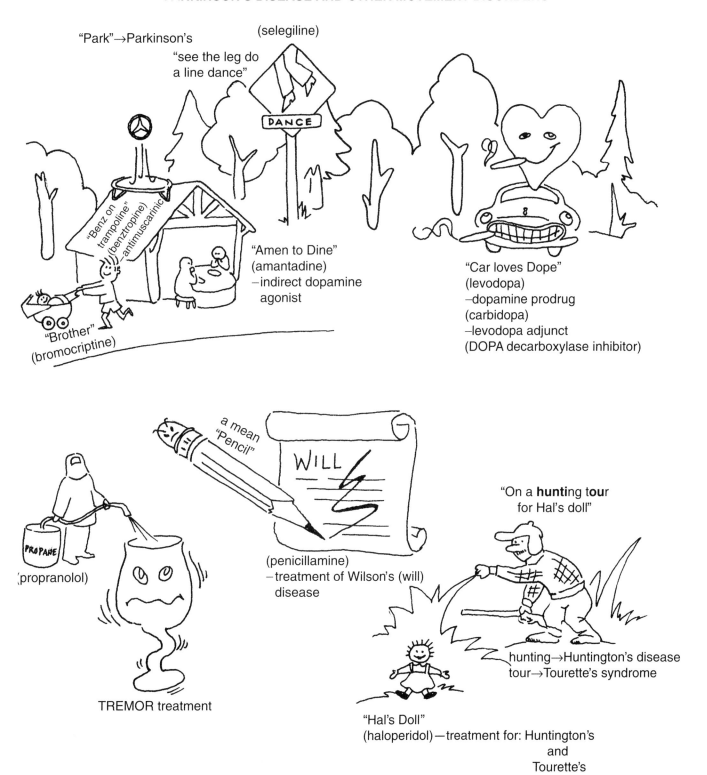

"Park"→Parkinson's

(selegiline)

"see the leg do a line dance"

DANCE

"Benz on trampoline" (benztropine) —antimuscarinic

"Amen to Dine" (amantadine) —indirect dopamine agonist

"Car loves Dope" (levodopa) —dopamine prodrug (carbidopa) —levodopa adjunct (DOPA decarboxylase inhibitor)

"Brother" (bromocriptine)

PROPANE

(propranolol)

TREMOR treatment

a mean "Pencil"

WILL

(penicillamine) —treatment of Wilson's (will) disease

"On a **hunt**ing **tour** for Hal's doll"

hunting→Huntington's disease tour→Tourette's syndrome

"Hal's Doll" (haloperidol)—treatment for: Huntington's and Tourette's

NOTES

ANTIEPILEPTIC DRUGS

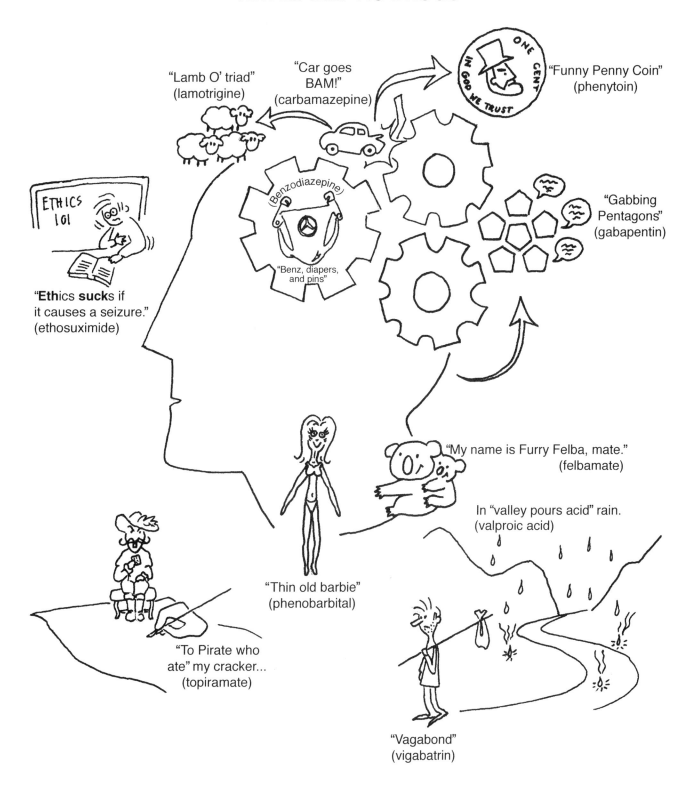

NOTES

PHARMACOLOGY OF ALCOHOLS

Ethanol is used in methanol and ethylene glycol poisoning because it is a preferred substrate of ADH, therefore slowing formation of toxic metabolites.

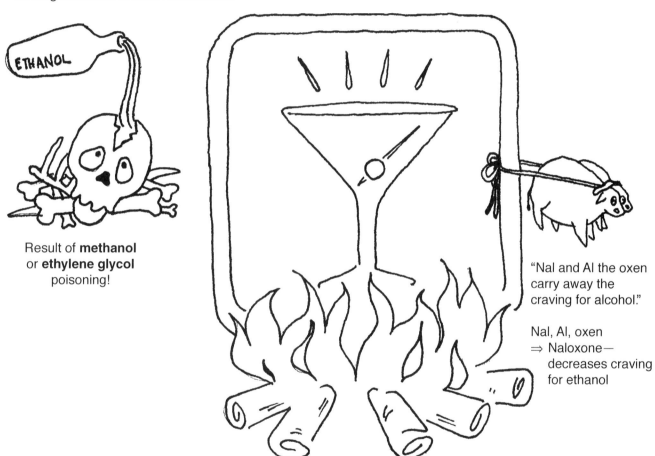

Result of **methanol** or **ethylene glycol** poisoning!

"Nal and Al the oxen carry away the craving for alcohol."

Nal, Al, oxen
⇒ Naloxone— decreases craving for ethanol

"Alcoholics dislike fire."

dislike fire
⇒ disulfiram—inhibits aldehyde dehydrogenase which converts **acetaldehyde** to acetic acid

NOTES

ANTIHYPERLIPIDEMIC

HMG–CoA reductase inhibitors
Simmons⇒**sim**vastatin
loves⇒**lov**astatin
praise⇒**pra**vastatin
flush⇒**flu**vastatin
2 = Type II
3 = Type III
2–5 = Types II–V
cholestra⇒**cholest**yramine
• binds fatty acids
clofib⇒**clofib**rate
• inhibits fatty acid absorption⇒Abs
gem⇒**gem**fibrozil
• raises HDL
nice⇒**ni**acin
probing⇒**prob**ucol

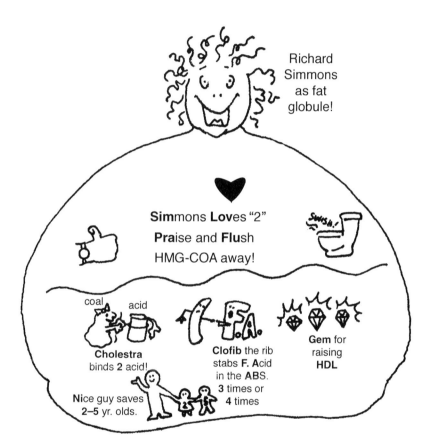

THE LIPID GLOBULE ASKS **PRO**BING QUESTIONS.

INDEX